Drs. Hannah and Abraham Stone's

A MARRIAGE MANUAL

*The famous guide to sex and marriage
recommended by doctors and educators*

NEW EDITION, REVISED BY

Dr. Gloria Stone Aitken
*Staff Physician, Willets Health Center, Douglass College,
Rutgers University and*

Dr. Aquiles J. Sobrero
Director, Margaret Sanger Research Bureau

SIMON AND SCHUSTER • NEW YORK

Contents

tomy). Sterilization of the Female. Abortions. Legal
and Illegal Abortions. Social and Medical Aspects of
Abortion.

Marriage. Premature Ejaculation. Causes of Male Frigidity and Impotence. Genital Disproportion. Masturbation. Masturbation and Sexual Adjustment. Homosexuality. Homosexuality and Marriage.

Publisher's Foreword

The long and distinguished publishing history of *A Marriage Manual* is a source of pride to its publishers, tempered only by regret that Dr. Hannah Stone and Dr. Abraham Stone are no longer living to observe the continuing impact that their wise and helpful book has had throughout the world.

From its initial publication in 1935 it was obvious that the book filled a long-felt need. In an era when sex and marriage were not as widely discussed as they are today, it was not easy for young couples to obtain accurate and well-presented information about a subject that was naturally of interest to them. It was in fact a taboo subject in many circles. It is all the more tribute to the authors that they approached their task with directness and frankness. They were concerned only with presenting as clearly and fully as possible the information that they knew, from their long experience as physicians and marriage counselors, was needed by men and women of all ages. Their skill and expertise were combined with a wise and tasteful humanitarianism that raised the book above controversy.

From the very beginning the book found a wide audience in this country. In 1942 a British edition was published and well received, and since then *A Marriage Manual* has been made available in translation to a broad readership in the following countries: Sweden, Denmark, Finland, France, Germany, Israel, Italy, Poland, Brazil, Spain, Czechoslovakia, Yugoslavia (in Slovene as well as Serbo-Croat) and India (in Bengali, Hindi and Urdu).

When a thorough revision of *A Marriage Manual* was made in 1951, letters from readers all over the world contributed new questions or pointed out places where amplification was needed.

The present revision has been ably executed by the daughter of the original authors, Dr. Gloria Stone Aitken, who is herself a physician with Willets Health Center, Douglass College, Rutgers University, and Dr. Aquiles J. Sobrero, a successor to the Doctors Stone in his association with the Margaret Sanger Research Bureau. Their additions make the work contemporary with the newest findings in the related fields of marriage, family planning and birth control. But the subject of the book is in many aspects a timeless one, presenting, as the authors said in their foreword to the first edition, "the essential facts of mating and reproduction." It is a testimony to Dr. Hannah Stone and Dr. Abraham Stone that so much of their original work remains because it could not be improved upon. It is as clear, fresh and pertinent today as when it was written.

Foreword to the First Edition

IN WRITING this book it has been our object to present in a realistic and concrete manner and in simple, nontechnical language the essential facts of mating and reproduction. For many years we have had the opportunity in lectures and consultations to discuss with men and women their problems of sex and marriage. During the course of our work, we have become familiar with the practical and intimate sexual and marital problems that confront the average individual. This book is based largely upon the results of these experiences and is an attempt to meet the general need for more adequate information concerning the factors of human sex and reproduction.

A Marriage Manual is written in the form of hypothetical consultations between a physician and a young couple about to be married. In reality it does represent a composite record of many thousands of pre- and post-marital consultations—at the Marriage Consultation Centers of the Labor Temple and the Community Church, at the Birth Control Clinical Research Bureau of New York, and elsewhere. We have adopted the dialogue style because we felt that it lent itself more readily to a vivid presentation of the questions and discussions, and because it appeared to be most suitable for a graphic portrayal of the subject matter.

Our aim has been to deal mainly with the individual aspect of sex contact rather than with the social, ethical or moral problems of sex conduct. As such, this volume is offered primarily as a practical guide to sex and marriage. We have dealt at some length and detail with the structure and functions of the human sex organs because we feel that an intelligent union should be based on an understanding of the biological processes involved. We have also emphasized particularly the technique of the sexual relation and the problems of birth control because it has been our experience that an appreciation of the sex factors in marriage and reliable contraceptive information are essential for a well-adjusted and satisfactory marital union.

Though it may appear from the contents that some parts were written by one or the other of us, we have, as a matter of fact, made no attempt to divide the subject between us, but have written all of it jointly. It has been our custom for many years to exchange our medical experiences, impressions and observations and to discuss and analyze the various problems that have come to our attention. Hence all the material included represents the result of the experiences and viewpoints of both of us.

DR. HANNAH M. STONE
DR. ABRAHAM STONE

Drs. Hannah and Abraham Stone's

A MARRIAGE MANUAL

CHAPTER I

FITNESS FOR MARRIAGE

We are about to be married, Doctor, and we have come to you for a general consultation. We feel we need some information and advice before our marriage, and we have many questions to ask.

It certainly is a good idea to have such a consultation before marriage, and I shall, of course, be glad to give you whatever information I can. An understanding of the basic physical, psychological and social factors involved in marriage is definitely a great help toward a more satisfactory adjustment. But first tell me if there are any specific problems which concern you.

No, we have no particular problems, but we just feel that we know too little about marriage in general.

I suppose you have already read some books on the subject.

Very few. In fact, we were going to ask you to recommend them to us.

As we go along I shall mention many books that may interest you. Before we proceed, however, has either of you had a physical examination lately?

No, not for some time. That is really one of the reasons for our visit. We have heard a great deal about fitness for marriage, and we have been wondering what this means.

Very well, I shall arrange for both of you to be examined later. However, if you were seriously interested in the question of your fitness for marriage, you should not have waited until this late date.

By now, I presume, all your plans and arrangements have already been made, and it would probably be almost impossible to change them. To determine fitness for marriage it is really necessary to make a rather thorough study of the family background, the past and present health record, and the general physical condition of the individual. This should preferably be done some time before the final steps are taken.

The Objects of Marriage

We realize that it is rather late for us to ask about our fitness now. We come from pretty good stock, and neither of us has had any serious illness, so we somehow assumed that we were well. Are there any special standards of fitness for marriage, Doctor?

There really are no absolute norms or criteria of suitability for marriage. As in other fields, fitness implies the ability to meet the necessary requirements or purposes. The standards of fitness, therefore, depend upon what we consider the objects of marriage to be.

Men and women may marry for any number of individual reasons. Basically, however, they seek in marriage three main objectives: a stable, permanent association based on mutual affection, on love and companionship; the freedom and privilege of a sexual relationship; and the establishment of a home and a family. Love and companionship, sexual intimacy and procreation are, then, in our culture at least, the main motives for marriage.

Companionship

In our case we have decided to get married because—well, because we are in love, and marriage seemed the natural thing. It will give us, we felt, a fuller sense of belonging to each other and make it possible for us to share our lives more intimately.

Quite so. A man and a woman who love each other, who feel a deep mutual attraction, who have many interests, tastes, and ideals in common will after a while want to make their association secure and stable. They will want to live together, to share their experiences, to be assured of lasting companionship. Under present social and legal conditions this type of relationship can be achieved only through marriage.

Mating

Furthermore, they will also want to live together in a physical sense. Love is a mixture of sentiment and sensuality, and the sexual relation is a fundamental factor in marriage. Where a strong attraction exists there will also be the desire for a close physical intimacy, and marriage provides the social, legal, and moral sanctions for a sexual relationship.

Reproduction

Biologically, again, the object of marriage is not to legalize a sexual union, but rather to insure the survival of the species and of the race. From this point of view, marriage is not merely a sexual relationship, but a parental association. It is the union of a male and a female for the production and care of offspring, and reproduction is therefore another fundamental object of marriage.

Economic Fitness

What about the economic factor, Doctor? Doesn't that also play an important part in marriage?

Yes, you are quite right. The economic factor has played an important role in the evolution of marriage and the family, and it is still a major factor in marriage today. In every human society, until recently at least, man has been the provider and woman the preparer. Economic ability, especially on the part of the man, has generally been regarded as one of the most important social standards of fitness for marriage. In many societies, strength, endurance, and the ability to provide for the family are essential marital qualifications. In his *History of Human Marriage,* Westermarck reports that among many primitive tribes a young man first had to prove his skill and courage before he was allowed to choose a wife. Among certain natives of South Africa, for example, no young man was permitted to marry before he had killed some big game, such as a jaguar. If he killed five jaguars, he had a right to more than one wife. Among certain Eskimo tribes, a young man could claim his bride only after he had proved by his skill in hunting that he could support not only a wife and children but his parents-in-law as well.

At present, of course, no such feats of valor are expected of the young man, nor do parents assume that they will be supported by their prospective son-in-law. Today the combined economic skills of both husband and wife are sometimes necessary to insure their own support. Nevertheless, a man's ability to meet the economic needs of a home and a family is still of prime importance in marriage, and economic fitness for marriage must, of course, receive due consideration.

Would you say, then, Doctor, that a couple should postpone marriage until the husband is able to support the family?

No, not necessarily. I do not believe that it is always advisable to postpone marriage until the man is able to provide fully for a family. Young people reach physiological maturity many years before they can attain economic security; the gap seems to be constantly widening, and often it is unwise to wait for complete financial independence. Furthermore, education in today's world of specialization requires such a lengthy period of, if not expensive, at least nonremunerative endeavor that a young man may be well into his thirties before he can begin to make a living. In these circumstances the wife may have to work to support them both. In other cases, when the wife also is obtaining an advanced education, financial assistance from the parents may be the most advisable solution if the parents are able and willing to help.

The important consideration is not whether the man has the ability to support a family at the time of marriage, but whether he is working productively toward achieving that ability and is developing a sound potential.

But wouldn't a marriage on such a basis mean a delay in the raising of a family? This really applies to our own case, Doctor. We are both looking forward to having children, but we'd rather not have any until we are in a position to provide for their care and their needs ourselves, and this may not be possible for some time.

This is a problem which confronts many young couples today.

Most young people can marry only on the understanding that the coming of children will be voluntarily delayed until they are ready to plan for a family. That is why adequate information on the best methods available for the prevention of conception should be given at the time of marriage to every couple desiring such information. Eventually, of course, you will, like most couples, want to have children, and you will then plan your family accordingly.

But let us return to the question of physical and psychological fitness for marriage. If the basic motives for marriage are love and the achievement of a secure and lasting companionship, sexual intimacy and procreation, then a man and a woman, if they are to make a good marriage, should be emotionally stable and mature, they should have normal sexual capacities, and they should be sound enough physically and eugenically to have children.

Emotional Fitness

What is emotional fitness for marriage, Doctor? Is it possible to tell whether one is emotionally fit for marriage?

This brings up the question of emotional maturity and what it implies, and I intend to discuss this point with you more fully at a later time. In general, there are people who are mentally and temperamentally grown-up or mature enough to be able to make a satisfactory adjustment in marriage even under difficult circumstances, and there are others who, because of their temperament, their disposition, their lack of maturity, are unable to make a successful marriage under any circumstances. An individual's personality, therefore, plays a very important part in the ability to establish a stable and happy relationship.

But is it not mainly a question of compatibility between husband and wife?

Not necessarily. When I speak of emotional fitness for marriage, I am not referring to the question of whether the two are compatible, but rather to the personalities of the individuals themselves. Let me tell you, as an example, about a couple I saw not long ago. It was the husband's third marriage. The first two had ended in divorce after constant domestic disagreements and conflicts which apparently could not be resolved. Now difficulties and dissensions were beginning to develop in the third marriage. After several interviews it became clear that the basis of the maladjustment in this case lay in the neurotic personality of the husband. He happened to have an exaggerated attachment to his mother, who had always dominated his life, an attachment from which he had not yet freed himself sufficiently to be able to enter fully into a new association.

Does an attachment to one's family usually prove a hindrance to satisfactory marriage?

On the contrary, an attachment to one's family is a normal outgrowth of a happy, loving family life, and this is the best preparation one can have for the formation of a happy marriage of one's own. In the case cited above there was an excessive degree of attachment and dependency. It is obvious, however, that after marriage a new understanding must enter into the family relationship. The new couple then should be emotionally free from parental domination, and they should be able to strike a sound balance between their loyalty to their respective parents and their relation to each other. "Therefore shall a man leave his father and his mother," says the Bible, "and shall cleave unto his wife." When a man and woman marry they should be able to break away from the original unit and build up a new unit for themselves.

Parental overattachment is, of course, only one of the reasons why some people are not emotionally ready for marriage. There are many other causes. There are men and women with neurotic or even psychotic personalities who may not be able to achieve a satisfactory marital adjustment with any mate. There are people, for instance, who are compulsive, or obsessive, who try to escape reality by resorting to alcohol or drugs, who have conscious or unconscious homosexual tendencies or other forms of sexual deviations. Under such circumstances the question of their emotional or psychological fitness for marriage must be seriously considered.

Sexual Fitness

When you spoke of normal sexual capacities in relation to physical fitness for marriage, Doctor, what specifically did you mean?

I was referring primarily to the physical ability of a person to enter into the sexual relationship. This is a problem which applies mainly to the man, although women too may suffer from physical or emotional disabilities which affect their sexual fitness. Inadequate potency on the part of the man, however, is a much more frequent condition, and one suffering from this disorder may be unable to consummate the physical union in marriage. It is a serious mistake for anyone who is sexually inadequate to marry without first having his disability corrected, or at least without receiving competent medical advice. As a matter of fact, Hindu lawmakers decreed over a thousand years ago that before marriage "a man must undergo an examination with regard to his virility." Only after the fact of his virility had been established beyond doubt was he privileged to marry.

If a man has never had sexual relations, is there any way of determining whether he is potent or not?

Only indirectly, of course. Normally every man, even though he may never have had any actual sex relations, has had some kind of sexual experience. In his study of the sex behavior of the American male, Kinsey found that practically all men engage in some form of sexual activity, which usually begins in childhood or adolescence. A man is, therefore, usually fairly well aware of the degree of his sexual adequacy. At times, it is true, a man may encounter unexpected difficulties after marriage, but, as a rule, he does have some knowledge beforehand of his sexual capacity or incapacity.

Reproductive Fitness

If a man is sexually potent, Doctor, does it also mean that he is capable of having children?

No, not necessarily. Potency—that is, the ability to have sexual relations—is not the same as fertility, which is the ability to reproduce. A man may be highly potent and yet not be fertile, or he may be very fertile and not be sexually potent. We shall discuss this point at length when we talk of the problems of reproduction.

How, then, can you judge fitness to have children?

Fitness for reproduction implies the ability to beget healthy children. It means freedom from any infirmity or disease which would make procreation physically or eugenically impossible or inadvisable.

Is it possible to know in advance whether a man or a woman will be able to have children?

If a fairly fresh specimen of the man's seminal fluid is obtained and examined microscopically, his fertility can be determined with considerable accuracy. Whenever there is any doubt concerning a man's fertility, as in the presence of some congenital abnormality, or an injury or disease of the reproductive organs, such an examination of the semen should certainly be made prior to marriage. Some even advocate a routine study of a man's seminal fluid as part of the general premarital examination.

It is also possible to estimate to some extent the fertility of the woman, but there are no methods available as yet to establish with certainty whether a particular couple will be fertile together. By a medical examination, however, a doctor can often determine whether any condition is present which might make procreation difficult or impossible.

Rh Factor

We've heard so much about the Rh factor in the blood. What bearing does it have upon a couple's ability to have children?

In 1940 a special substance was discovered in the blood which was named the Rh factor, after the Rhesus monkey, in which this blood factor was first noted. It was found that eighty-five per cent of all white persons carry this Rh factor in their blood and are thus "Rh positive," while fifteen per cent lack this factor and are "Rh negative." In peoples of other races, Indians, Chinese or Negroes, the percentage of Rh-positive persons is considerably higher.

When an Rh-positive man marries an Rh-negative woman, which happens in about thirteen per cent of white marriages, the children of such a marriage may develop a condition known as erythroblastosis, which is characterized mainly by anemia, jaundice and swellings of the body. Fortunately only about one in twenty-seven of these children is so affected. The condition is due to the action of substances developed by the mother, called antibodies, that act against the red blood cells of the unborn baby. In recent years much work has been done in this field, including the development of tests such as prenatal analysis of the mother's amniotic fluid—the fluid within the bag of water—which indicates with some accuracy the status of the fetus. Until a few years ago, severely affected infants often died before birth. Today, preterm delivery and sometimes intrauterine transfusions or exchange transfusions immediately after birth save many previously unsalvageable babies.

Reports emanating from Germany in 1966 and recent studies in this country hold the brightest promise for this whole problem. It has been shown by several researchers that mothers may be immunized against Rh-positive antigen with a special preparation of gamma globulin. These mothers never develop the Rh antibodies, and their offspring are unaffected. If this approach is found to be as effective as early tests indicate, Rh incompatibility will be another conquered disease.

Health of the Husband

Has a person's general health any relation to fitness for marriage?

Good health is, naturally, a desirable asset under all circumstances, and a "bad liver" may spoil even an ideal romance. Yet, generally speaking, perfect health is not essential for marriage. Suppose a man had scarlet fever in his childhood which left him with a chronic kidney ailment, or he had rheumatic fever at one time which had affected his heart—this does not necessarily bear upon his fitness for marriage. It may influence his earning capacity, his prospects for the future, the duration of his life, or even his general disposition and reactions, but it does not make him ineligible for marriage or incapable of making a fine husband. We have seen any number of marriages that were entirely happy and satisfactory in spite of the fact that one or the other of the couple was not in perfect physical condition. However, when a chronic physical handicap does exist, it is well that the couple should know it beforehand, so that the situation may be clearly understood and voluntarily accepted by both. Every now and then serious marital difficulties result from the fact that either the husband or the wife had failed to disclose before marriage the existence of a chronic disability.

Health of the Wife

This is especially important when the woman is suffering from some chronic disorder which would make childbearing hazardous for her. To a woman with a bad heart, for instance, a pregnancy may constitute a considerable risk to health and even to life. The presence of such a condition should be discussed in advance of the marriage, so that there may be a mutual understanding of the possibilities involved and an opportunity to make the needed physical and emotional adjustments.

But suppose a person can't or shouldn't have children for one reason or another. Should he never marry?

No, not necessarily. Couples do marry in spite of the fact that they know beforehand that they never can or should have children, and such marriages are often quite successful. There are other factors which may influence a man or a woman to marry—factors which outweigh the inability to beget children. In such circumstances, however, both should know of the condition beforehand and enter the marriage with such knowledge and understanding in mind.

In the main, a man and a woman who are deeply and maturely in love with each other will want to be married even though the marriage may not be able to satisfy all their needs and expectations. Often they will find that many of their fears and anxieties about their future relationship turn out to be quite baseless.

Eugenic Fitness

Is there any way of telling beforehand whether a couple's children will be healthy?

This brings up the question of eugenics and eugenic fitness for marriage. Naturally the man and woman who marry expect that their children will be born sound in mind and body. While there are no tests by which the physical or mental qualities of the future child can be foretold, if both parents are healthy and free from any transmissible disease, and if there is no family history of any hereditary abnormality, there is every reason to assume that their children will be normal. If, however, either one of them suffers from some physical or mental ailment which might be transmitted to offspring, or if there is a hereditary defect in the family, the possibilities should be carefully considered and competent advice obtained before marriage.

What kinds of abnormalities is it possible for children to inherit, Doctor?

The human body is a highly complex organism, and it is possible for many kinds of defects to be inherited. The great majority of children, however, are fortunately born free from such defects. The inherited defects that do occur include various types of structural abnormalities, diseases of the blood, of the nervous system or of the glands, mental ailments or deficiencies, blindness, deafness and a number of other rarer disorders. Similar defects and diseases may, however, also result from environmental and nonhereditary factors, and it is therefore necessary to establish in each instance separately whether the condition was inherited or acquired.

The Mechanism of Heredity

How are hereditary conditions passed on from one generation to another?

Parents transmit to their children a vast number of factors which go to make up the inherited physical and mental characteristics of the individual. As you may know, every human being arises out of the union of two microscopic cells, the sperm of the male and the egg of the female. In these minute cells are certain bodies called chromosomes, which are in turn made up of a very large number of individual units, technically known as genes. These genes are the physical elements which determine the hereditary characteristics of the child—the shape of his features, the color of his eyes, of his hair, of his skin, and other physical details of his body. They also have an influence on the child's intelligence, as well as, indirectly perhaps, on his personality and emotional characteristics.

Chromosomes and Genes

The genes may be present in an enormous number of combinations within the chromosomes. When you consider that each parent contributes twenty-three chromosomes to the fertilized egg, you can see that the number of chance combinations of genes in a given individual is almost infinite. It has been mathematically calculated that there are some sixteen million possible combinations of hereditary traits from each parent. The chance of the same combination of genes in an egg and sperm occurring twice is one in three hundred trillion. Geneticists state that there have not been two identical men. The occurrence of identical twins is a different matter altogether and one that we will discuss at another time.

If the color of the eyes is inherited, Doctor, why is it that sometimes when both the father and the mother have brown eyes the child's eyes are blue?

This difference in eye-color distribution is a good illustration of the mechanism of heredity. Each child inherits two sets of genes, one from the father and one from the mother, but the characteristics of the child will depend not only upon the types of genes it inherits but also upon the way the genes will combine. In eye color, for instance, if the child happens to inherit a gene for brown eyes from the father and another for brown from the mother, his eyes will be brown and he will be able to transmit genes only for brown eyes to his children. If he inherits genes for blue eyes from both parents, his eyes will be blue and he will be able to transmit blue eyes only. If, however, he receives a gene for brown from the father and one for blue from the mother, his own eyes will be brown, because it happens that the "brown" gene dominates or masks the "blue" one, but he will also carry a gene for blue in his chromosomes and he will be able to transmit to his offspring genes either for brown or for blue eyes. In the case you mentioned, the parents, presumably, each have genes both for brown and for blue, and their children may, therefore, inherit either brown or blue eyes. Please understand that this is a rather oversimplified explanation, for even the color of the eyes is determined in a much more complex manner. It serves, however, to illustrate the general pattern of heredity.

Heredity and Environment

Are mental and personal traits also inherited in the same way? Doesn't environment play a large part?

The inheritance of mental and temperamental qualities has been a source of much controversy. Early eugenists maintained that a child's intelligence and personality were determined almost entirely by heredity. Later the "behaviorists" claimed that environment—education, training, early experiences, and conditioning—was almost entirely responsible for making children what they were or what they developed into. Today the belief is becoming general that heredity and environment constantly interact, and that the two can never be clearly separated since environmental differences start even before birth. The noted biologist Jennings, in his book *The Biological Basis of Human Nature,* ably analyzes the relative influence of environment and heredity, and concludes that intelligence, behavior, temperament, and disposition can be modified by either of these. Even identical twins with exactly the same heredity, for instance, will, if placed in different environments, show some variations in mental development, personality and character. In other words, marked differences between individuals can be produced by varying either the heredity or the environment.

The relation of heredity to environment is perhaps most simply expressed as the relation of the seed to the soil, a comparison which has frequently been made. The seed has potentialities to develop into a certain type of plant, but whether these potentialities will be realized will depend to a very large degree upon the kind of soil into which it is planted; in poor soil it will be stunted, in good soil it will develop to its fullest capacities. On the other hand, no matter how good the soil, it can only bring out the qualities which were already present in the seed at the time it was sown. Nature and nurture constantly interact, and they are perhaps equally important in determining the character of an individual.

Congenital Defects

If a child is born with some defect, does it always mean that it is inherited?

Not necessarily. Certain defects or diseases may be acquired by the baby during the period of growth in its mother's womb, or even at the time it is being born, and such defects are not inherited. We should distinguish clearly between a condition which is congenital —that is, which is merely present at birth—and one which is hereditary. It has recently been found, for instance, that if a woman becomes infected with German measles and possibly other viral diseases during the first three months of pregnancy, the virus of the disease may pass from the mother to the growing child within her and cause either an abortion or—if the fetus is carried to term —malformations of organs such as the eye, the ear and the heart. Such a condition is congenital. The child is born with it, but it is not hereditary and will not be passed by inheritance to a subsequent generation. Similarly, if a mother becomes infected with chicken pox during pregnancy the virus may infect the child during its intra-uterine life and the child will be born with chicken pox. The disease is not an inherited one, however, even though it is present at birth. A hereditary factor is one which is inherent in the reproductive cells of the parents and which is therefore transmitted to the child as a very part of its constitutional makeup at the time the egg is initially fertilized by the sperm.

In the 1960s there was a tragic epidemic of birth defects that was traced to the use of a tranquilizer drug, thalidomide, during early pregnancy. Since that time more stringent tests on the effect of drugs on the unborn are being required, and it has become a general rule that absolutely no unnecessary drugs should be taken by pregnant women. These defects, again, are not hereditary.

Acquired and Inherited Defects

Is it possible to tell whether a physical abnormality in a child is inherited or not?

That will depend upon the particular disorder. We must distinguish clearly between ailments that are inherited and those that are acquired. Acquired disabilities are not familial. One may, for instance, develop a certain deformity as a result of an attack of infantile paralysis, but a deformity of this type would not be hereditary and would not be transmitted to the children. Or one may become deaf because of an injury or infection of the ear, but this form of deafness is not transmissible.

Certain physical abnormalities are, however, definitely inherited. Recently, for example, I saw a child with six fingers on each hand. The child's father and grandmother had a similar abnormality, and it was obviously a case of an inherited condition. The same is true of certain types of disorders of the eyes and ears, of bleeding tendencies, and of other defects which appear in successive generations of a family, and which are caused by defective genes. More important, even, is the fact that it is possible to inherit or to transmit a constitutional weakness which makes the individual more susceptible to a particular disease. Thus a predisposition to certain types of disorders can be transmitted by the parents, but whether the condition will actually develop in the child will depend upon later environmental factors.

Transmission of Defective Genes

If the parents are entirely well and have never had any sickness, is it still possible for them to pass on some family defect to their children?

Unfortunately, it is. An individual may be entirely normal himself and yet carry a defective gene within him, as one may, for instance, have brown eyes, as we saw, and nevertheless carry within him a gene for blue eyes. The same applies to other characteristics, both normal and abnormal. As a matter of fact, the existence of defective genes in normal people and the possibility of their transmission constitutes one of the basic problems of eugenics.

Can a person know whether he carries defective genes?

There is no definite way of determining the presence of any hidden or potential defect in an individual who is normal himself. In a general way, though, if a couple has no serious abnormality and if there is no record of any hereditary disease in their families, they may assume that they will have normal children. If both of them are well, and there is a history, let us say, of some hereditary defect in one of the families, the possible chances of transmission will depend upon the type of the disease, the manner of its inheritance, the number and nearness of the relatives afflicted, and many other factors.

What about tuberculosis, Doctor? If one or both of the parents have the disease, are their children apt to inherit it?

New drugs have greatly altered both the incidence and the course of this disease, and the outlook today is far more encouraging than it used to be. The question of marriage would depend upon the extent of the infection and the individual circumstances. In early or arrested cases marriage is not inadvisable, for with proper care the disease can be kept permanently in check. In the more advanced cases the situation is more serious and each instance must be decided separately. There are several factors which have to be taken into consideration: the chance of early incapacity and invalidism; the emotional reactions and adjustments; the possibility of infecting the partner; and, in the case of the woman, the question of childbearing, for a pregnancy may seriously aggravate an existing tuberculosis and endanger the patient's life.

Cancer and Heredity

Is there any hereditary factor in cancer? Is one more apt to develop the disease if there have been cases in the family?

How cancer develops is still a baffling problem, but any direct inheritance of the common forms of the disease has not yet been established. There is a possibility that a somewhat increased susceptibility to cancer, or at least to certain forms of it, may be transmitted to the child. The evidence for this is, however, certainly not yet clear enough to restrain anyone from marrying or from having children, even if the disease is present in one or more members of a family. Furthermore, there is always the possibility that a cure for cancer may be found in the not far distant future.

Inherited Susceptibilities

What about susceptibility to other diseases?

Even though a predisposition to some disease may be inherited, the individual may never develop the disease, or it may be avoided by adequate care. Hay fever, for instance, a condition caused by a sensitivity to certain pollens, is a good example. There is considerable evidence that a susceptibility to hay fever may be inherited, but obviously if one happens to live in a district free from the offending pollen, he will never develop hay fever even if he does inherit a predisposition to it.

This is true of quite a number of diseases. In his interesting book on heredity, Scheinfeld points out that this applies in some measure to rheumatic fever. This condition usually develops in childhood, and is more likely to occur in some families than in others, presumably because of inherited weaknesses. It is dependent upon some reaction of the body to infection with a certain type of streptococcus. This does not mean, however, that a child who inherits such a susceptibility will of necessity develop the disease. It is much more apt to appear under conditions of poverty and overcrowding, and its development, therefore, depends to a large extent upon the environment in which the child is brought up.

Gonorrhea and Heredity

Are the venereal diseases hereditary?

There are two main venereal diseases to be considered, gonorrhea and syphilis, and each presents its own special problems. Gonorrhea is a local infection of the sex and urinary organs. Only rarely do the germs of the disease enter the bloodstream and spread to other parts of the body. In any event, it is not transmitted to the offspring as an inherited infection.

But people are always saying that if the parents have gonorrhea the children may be born diseased.

Yes, a newborn child may develop gonorrhea, but not because the disease is inherited. The child contracts it by being infected with the germs at the time of its birth. If the gonorrhea germs are present in the birth canal of the mother, the infant may become infected during its passage through the canal. The germs may lodge in the eyes of the infant and produce a very serious inflammation which may result in blindness. That is the reason why the eyes of the baby are treated by the doctor soon after its birth with an antiseptic solution as a routine measure. This application has proved to be an effective prophylactic against the transmission of the disease to the newborn, and has greatly reduced the amount of infant blindness resulting from this infection.

Syphilis and Heredity

What about syphilis, Doctor? Isn't this disease transmitted from parents to their children?

Syphilis presents an entirely different problem. First of all, it is not a local disease like gonorrhea, but a generalized infection. It usually starts as a local sore or ulceration on the genitals or other parts of the body, but from there the germs soon enter the bloodstream and are carried through the entire system. They may lodge in any organ and produce serious consequences, sometimes, in fact, many years after the first appearance of the infection. If not adequately treated, the disease may be transmitted to the offspring, in the same way that chicken pox is transmitted to the fetus, as we discussed before. Syphilis is rarely transmitted to the fetus before the fifth month of pregnancy, and an infected mother therefore has adequate time to obtain treatment to protect her baby. What happens is that after the fifth month of pregnancy the germs pass from the mother to the developing child and infect it with the disease. The embryo may die early as a result of the infection; or it may continue to live for several months and die just before birth, the pregnancy ending in a miscarriage or stillbirth; or, if the fetus is strong enough to survive the initial attack, the infant will be born with the infection present in its body. In other words, syphilis in the newborn is a congenital rather than a hereditary disease.

Venereal Diseases and Marriage

How safe is it for someone who has had a venereal disease to marry and bear children?

Each case must be decided individually. Certainly no one who has had a venereal infection should marry without being assured by a competent physician that he can no longer transmit the disease. Because of their prevalence and far-reaching consequences, the venereal diseases constitute a real problem in relation to fitness for marriage. However, present-day methods of treating these diseases have greatly lessened their danger and the chances of their being transmitted to future children.

Can either gonorrhea or syphilis be completely cured?

Yes. Development of modern methods for the treatment of both gonorrhea and syphilis, including the use of penicillin and other agents, has, in fact, made fairly rapid cures possible. Gonorrhea, for instance, if treated in its early stages, can be cured within a week by large doses of the proper antibiotics.

Syphilis is a much more serious condition and more difficult to cure. It is not always easy to rid the body of this infection, and it may require repeated treatment before a patient can be made free of the disease. Nevertheless, it is the opinion of most authorities that this can be accomplished in the majority of cases. The sooner treatment is begun after the onset of the disease, the better the chances of a permanent cure. If the patient has received active treatment and has been entirely free from any evidence of the disease he or she need not fear transmitting the infection to the spouse or offspring. It is a discouraging fact, however, that although there was a steady decline in the incidence of venereal disease after the advent of penicillin, this trend has been reversed since 1958. In 1957 there were 216,476 reported cases of gonorrhea in the United States, and in 1964 this had risen to 291,598. The highest proportion of infectious venereal disease is among teenagers and young adults. In New Jersey, for instance, the syphilitic rate for the fifteen-to-nineteen-year-old group jumped from 7 cases per 100,000 in 1958 to almost 39 in 1963 and in the twenty-to-twenty-four-year-old group from 13 per 100,000 in 1958 to 107 in 1963.

Premarital Blood Tests

Don't most states now require a blood test for venereal disease before marriage?

Yes, persons suffering from a venereal disease in a communicable form are now forbidden by law to marry in most states. In New York, for example, a law was passed in 1938 requiring a premarital medical examination for syphilis, including a blood test, of all applicants for a marriage license. Before a license is issued, the applicant must submit a statement signed by a physician to the effect that he or she is free from syphilis in a stage which may become communicable. The statement must include a laboratory report showing that a blood test has been made within thirty days of the application for the marriage license. If more than thirty days elapse, another blood test is required.

Similar laws requiring premarital blood tests, and in most cases medical examinations for the presence of syphilis, have now been enacted in most of our states. Some states also require a physical examination for gonorrhea. These laws are useful because, aside from actually preventing the marriage of infectious individuals, they create an awareness of the dangers of transmitting venereal diseases.

Prenatal Blood Tests

Incidentally, most states now also require a blood test for syphilis on every pregnant woman. The object is to detect the presence of the disease early in the pregnancy so that adequate treatment may be given in time to prevent the child from becoming infected. If sufficient treatment is received during pregnancy, the child will usually be born free from the infection.

Inherited Mental Abnormalities

Are mental diseases or abnormalities always inherited?

There is still a great deal of controversy as to the relative importance of hereditary and environmental factors, such as birth injuries, early experiences, emotional shocks, glandular disorders or general infections in the causation of mental disorders. Nevertheless, the consensus seems to be that at least in a certain percentage of psychoses, of epilepsy, feeble-mindedness and other types of mental disturbances, there is definite evidence of some hereditary tendency or defect.

Epilepsy

I know a family in which both parents are apparently entirely normal, yet one of the sons recently developed epilepsy. Could there be a question of inheritance in such a case?

The convulsions or fits which are characteristic of epilepsy may be either acquired or inherited. Injuries to the brain during birth, for instance, head injuries, especially during infancy or childhood, tumors, infectious diseases, allergic conditions—any of these may lead to the development of epileptic convulsions. These forms of epilepsy are, of course, not inherited and cannot be transmitted to a future generation.

There is, however, a type of epilepsy which is hereditary, but present medical opinion holds that the child does not actually inherit the disease itself but a predisposition to it. By means of a special operation it is possible to record and measure the pattern of the electrical waves produced by the activity of the nervous cells of the brain of an individual, and it has been established that the frequency and type of these waves are hereditary traits. In epileptics these brain waves show a peculiar irregularity, and these irregularities are often present in otherwise normal relatives of epileptics. Abnormal waves are regarded as indicative of an unstable brain activity, but some other environmental factor is required to produce an epileptic episode or fit. The chance that a child of an epileptic will also be epileptic is about one in forty. Some epileptics, therefore, may marry and bear children with safety, and others may not. A study of the brain waves may in some instances assist in advising epileptic families about parenthood.

Marriage Between Relatives

People say that near relatives should not marry because their children are apt to be abnormal. Is there any scientific basis for this idea?

The physical and mental qualities of offspring coming from first cousins or other near relatives are subject to the same laws of heredity which govern the children of nonrelatives. If the father and the mother are closely related, the chances of the child's inheriting the traits appearing in that family are very much increased. If these characteristics happen to be good, so much the better for the child; but if there happens to exist some physical or mental deficiency in the family, the child will be more likely to inherit the undesirable traits. In some families close intermarriage has produced brilliant offspring; in others it has perpetuated defective traits. Recently, for instance, I saw a young woman who was suffering from a hereditary form of deafness. Four of her brothers and one sister had a similar condition. Neither of the parents is deaf, but they were first cousins and there were several instances of hereditary deafness on both sides of the family. In this case, obviously, inbreeding tended to bring to the fore the family defect. Marriages between relatives, therefore, should be considered individually. In general, perhaps, such marriages should not be encouraged, but neither should they be prohibited.

Individual Eugenics

From a eugenic standpoint, Doctor, are there any standards one may follow in choosing a mate?

If one were to select a mate only on a eugenic basis, with the sole idea of insuring healthy offspring, one would naturally seek a person who is both physically and mentally healthy and whose family background is free from any hereditary defects. Few people, however, are at present willing to permit eugenic considerations to guide entirely the affairs of the heart. Cupid will not easily be replaced by a eugenic board, and, in view of our present limitation of genetic knowledge, perhaps it is just as well that this is so. Theoretically the best advice that can be given is to avoid marriage with someone who is afflicted with a serious transmissible defect, and refrain from marrying into a family that happens to possess the same kinds of bodily and mental hereditary weaknesses as one's own. To a couple in love eugenic considerations are not always the most important factor in planning a marriage, but they should be completely aware of the potential hazards to which their offspring might be subject. When the maternal and paternal genes are shuffled together in the new-formed child, the outlook for the child is apt to be much more favorable if the two sets come from different stocks and contain many divergent qualities. In the choice of a mate from a eugenic viewpoint, it is well also, of course, to give preference to one who comes from a family with desirable traits. In fact, one of the chief aims of the modern eugenic movement is the development of a positive eugenic consciousness.

Racial Eugenics

What program do the eugenists recommend, Doctor?

The purpose of eugenics is to breed a better human race. Francis Galton, the English scientist who founded the movement, maintained that most human differences are innate and inborn, and that it should therefore be possible to improve the human stock by breeding from the best. Some human beings, according to the eugenists, are physically and mentally superior, and others are inferior. The superior group, because of their greater foresight and higher standards, is limiting the number of its offspring, while those of the inferior group continue to multiply at a more rapid rate. To prevent the deterioration of the human race, they say, the superior people should be encouraged to have more children by making them conscious of their responsibilities and by giving them special social aids and privileges, while the reproduction of the socially inadequate should be discouraged by eugenic education and the provision of means for family limitation.

Doesn't that bring us back, though, to the problem of heredity and environment? Isn't social superiority or inferiority often as much a question of chance and opportunity as of hereditary qualities?

You are quite right. As long as the eugenists distinguish merely between people who are biologically sound or unsound, they are, I believe, well justified in their conclusions. Certainly individuals afflicted with serious hereditary deficiencies—the grossly abnormal, the feeble-minded, the psychotic—should be prevented from reproducing. When the eugenists, however, attempt to classify mankind into superior and inferior classes, into the better groups and the "socially inadequate" or the "social-problem" groups, their claims become subject to serious criticisms. Such a stratification of society may rest more on economic and social grounds than on actual biological differences. It is hardly possible, after all, to tell whether the people who today occupy the higher positions in society have reached their stations because of superior native endowments or because of some favorable environmental factors—better education, better opportunities, better connections, and so on. There can hardly be any doubt, in fact, that among the socially inadequate there are any number of individuals who might have attained greater social heights and been considered among the superiors, had they had a different economic, social and environmental background from the start. The majority of us probably have native capacities and potentialities which are never brought to the surface because of a lack of opportunity, and it is very likely that an improvement or change in economic and social conditions may result in a considerable regrouping of our social strata. Perhaps such an improvement may accomplish more for social advance than any system of strict eugenic selection which may be employed at the present time.

In their program to encourage marriage and reproduction among healthy individuals, the eugenists have, however, many valuable positive suggestions. They favor marriage grants to young persons, salary increases for married men, low-cost housing projects, adequate prenatal care, lower maternity costs, maternity leaves for working mothers. Such measures would make it easier for young people to marry and to bear and care for the children they desire.

We have had a rather long session today, and perhaps we had better postpone our further discussions for another time. In the meantime both of you will have your physical examinations. Before you go, however, I should like to give you the names of several books which you might read in connection with some of the subjects we were considering today and will consider in our future sessions.

Bibliography

Bowman, Henry A., *Marriage for Moderns,* 5th ed. McGraw-Hill, 1965.

Burgess, Ernest W., and Fishbein, Morris, M.D., eds., *Successful Marriage,* rev. ed. Doubleday, 1955.

Burgess, Ernest W., and Locke, Harvey J., *The Family,* 3rd ed. American Book Company, 1963.

Cavan, Ruth S., *The American Family,* 3rd ed. Crowell, 1963.

Cavanagh, John R., M.D., *Fundamental Marriage Counseling: A Catholic Viewpoint.* Bruce Publishing Company, 1963.

Christensen, Harold T., ed., *Handbook of Marriage and the Family.* Rand McNally, 1964.

Duvall, Evelyn Millis, *Love and the Facts of Life.* Association Press, 1963. Also in paperback.

——, *Why Wait till Marriage?* Association Press, 1965. Also in paperback.

——, and Hill, Reuben, *When You Marry,* rev. ed. Association Press, 1962.

Merrill, Francis E., *Society and Culture,* 3rd ed. Prentice-Hall, 1965.

Scheinfeld, Amram, *Your Heredity and Environment* (formerly *The New You and Heredity*). Lippincott, 1965.

Schur, Edwin M., ed., *The Family and the Sexual Revolution: Selected Readings.* Indiana University Press, 1964.

Thomas, John L., S.J., *Looking Toward Marriage.* Fides Publishers, 1964.

Westermarck, Edward, *Short History of Marriage.* College Library, 1926.

See also the comprehensive Bibliography at the back of the book for further titles, including some classic references no longer in print.

CHAPTER II

THE BIOLOGY
OF MARRIAGE

THE MALE SEX ORGANS

I am glad to let you know that the results of the examination and of the tests we took last time all proved to be satisfactory. Both of you are in good physical condition.

Thank you, Doctor. We've been well all along and didn't expect you to find anything wrong. Still, we're glad to get a clean bill of health. Neither of us had had a medical examination for some time.

Well, one really should have a general physical examination about once a year. In view of your coming marriage, I naturally paid special attention this time to the physical aspects of your fitness for marriage.

And now let us continue with our discussion. I should like to devote the time today to a review of the anatomy and physiology of the human reproductive system. How much do you know about the structure and function of the body?

We had some courses in school on the human body, but we don't remember very much of it now. I think you'd better assume that we know very little or nothing at all.

Very well. Naturally I shall not attempt to discuss with you the whole of human anatomy. I will limit myself to a brief review of the structure and functions of the male and female genital systems.

Anyone contemplating marriage ought to have some knowledge of sex and reproduction. This should really be a part of preparation for marriage.

The Role of the Male in Reproduction

The basis of sexual reproduction in nature is the union of the male and female sex cells, the sperm and the egg. The primary function of the sexes, therefore, as far as procreation is concerned, is the production of the respective sex cells. The role of the male, however, is not limited merely to the production of the sperm; he must, in addition, deposit them in a place where they will have the best chance of coming in contact with the female cells. In some of the lower forms of life no special provisions are made for this latter purpose. Among certain fishes and marine animals, for instance, both the male and the female when ready for reproduction deposit their sex cells directly in the waters. There is no direct contact between the two sexes, and the sperm and egg are left to meet by chance. In all the higher forms of life, however, special adaptations and organs have been evolved which serve to bring the spermatozoa, or sperm, close to or into the body of the female so that the union with the egg may be more fully assured. This is the case with the human species, where this meeting takes place within the genital tract of the female. In considering, therefore, the male sex organs, we may distinguish between those which are concerned primarily with the production of the sperm and those which serve to carry the sperm into the female.

Male Pelvis

To get a clearer picture of this mechanism, let us look at a diagram of the human male reproductive system (Figure1). It represents a side view of the organs which lie in the lower part of the abdomen below the waistline, that is, in the pelvis. The external genitals, too, are shown on this diagram.

To the right you can see the spinal column gradually tapering down. In front of it lies the lower part of the intestinal tract, the rectum, which communicates with the outside through the anus. In front of the rectum lies the bladder, a distensible, baglike organ which serves as a reservoir for the urine. Below the bladder and between it and the rectum are the several organs which form an accessory part of the reproductive system.

Kidneys, Ureters and Bladder

May I interrupt you, Doctor? I understand that the urine is formed by the kidneys. What is the relation of the kidneys to the bladder?

They are all a part of the urinary system. The urine is formed in the kidneys, but these lie higher up, one on each side of the abdomen, and are not shown on this diagram. Each kidney is connected with the bladder by a slender, delicate tube, the ureter. The urine is produced in the kidneys almost continuously and passes along the ureter, a few drops at a time, into the bladder. There it is stored until it is passed at urination through another tube, called the urethra, which leads from the bladder to the outside.

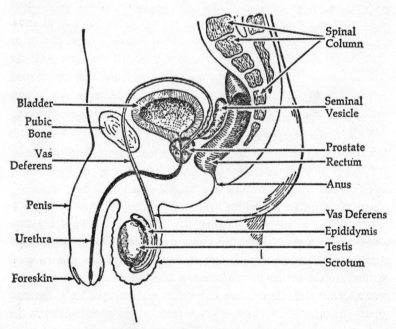

FIGURE 1. *Male Genital Organs (side view)*

*Is there any special connection between the urinary system and
the sexual organs?*

Yes, indeed, particularly in the man. Anatomically, the urinary
and the sexual apparatus are intimately related. For one thing, the
urethra, which is really the outlet of the urinary system, lies through
a great part of its length, as you see here, in the male copulative
organ, the penis, and it serves not merely for the passage of urine
but also for the transmission of the seminal fluid during an ejaculation. There are other organs, too, as we shall see later, which are
closely related to both systems.

The Seminal Fluid

What makes up the seminal fluid, Doctor?

The term "seminal fluid," or "semen," is applied to the material
discharged by the male during the ejaculation. The spermatozoa, or
sperm, constitute its most important element, but the bulk of this
fluid consists of the secretions from the other accessory sex glands,
the prostate and the seminal vesicles. During the ejaculation, all of
these secretions are brought together and make up the seminal discharge.

The Testes

The spermatozoa are formed in the testes—that is, male sex glands.
There is a right and a left testis, or testicle, each ovoid in shape
and about the size of an ordinary plum. They measure about one
and a half to two inches in length and about one inch in thickness,
but there is a considerable individual variation in different men.
The two testes are suspended in a special pouch called the scrotum,
which hangs downward behind the penis.

In addition to sperm formation, the testes also produce a special
secretion, or hormone, which is not a part of the seminal fluid. This
hormone is absorbed directly into the blood system and plays a very
significant role in the development of the individual's physical and
psychological male characteristics.

The Scrotum

Do the testicles change in size? I have been under the impression that they become larger or smaller at different times.

The testes do not change in size, but the scrotum, or the pouch in which they lie, is subject to expansions and contractions. In warm weather, for instance, or after a hot bath, the scrotum becomes relaxed and the testicles are lower; in cold weather, the muscles of the scrotum contract and bring the testes higher up nearer to the body, so that it may seem as if the glands have actually grown smaller in size. The object of this mechanism is to maintain the testes in the most suitable temperature, for they are very sensitive to heat and cold and require protection from environmental changes.

In fact, the temperature of the scrotum is a few degrees lower than that of the inside of the body, and this lowered temperature is essential for the proper functioning of the testes. It has been shown, for instance, that the application of heat or the insulation of the scrotum with a plastic tight suspender will cause considerable injury to the sperm-producing function of the testes, and may even result in sterility.

I have sometimes noticed that the left testicle seems to be lower than the right. Is there anything abnormal about that?

No, not at all. The left testicle is normally lower than the right, and is frequently somewhat larger in size.

Undescended Testes

A friend of mine was born with only one testicle. Does that happen often?

This is a condition which happens perhaps once in about five hundred men. Sometimes one and sometimes both of the testes are missing from the scrotum. In the embryo the testes lie within the abdominal cavity, but before birth they descend through a canal in the groin and lodge in the scrotum. In certain instances one or both of the glands may fail to come down, remaining either in the abdomen or in the groin. This condition is known as "undescended testicles" or cryptorchidism. Frequently the undescended testes come down of themselves around puberty due to their increased growth at this time, but sometimes it may become necessary to employ surgical means in order to lower them into the scrotum. Recent research has shown that the descent of the testes is dependent upon the action of a certain hormone which comes from the pituitary gland, and in many cases of undescended testes it is now possible to bring them down into the scrotum during the early years of the child's life by the administration of this pituitary hormone. If this is unsuccessful surgery may be employed.

When the testes do not descend into the scrotum at the proper time, does it have any special effect upon the man? Would it affect his sex life or his fitness for marriage?

If the testes remain undescended they may atrophy and lose their ability to produce sperm. Hence a man with undescended testes on both sides is very apt to be sterile. The internal secretions of the gland, however, do not seem to be affected, and the development of the physical and mental characteristics which are controlled by the testicular hormones proceed quite normally. Men with undescended testes are therefore quite normal physically and sexually, except that their seminal fluid does not contain any sperm. One descended testicle, however, is quite sufficient for the reproductive functions of the individual. Hence, if only one testicle is undescended, the sexual and procreative abilities are not affected in any way.

The Path of the Sperm from the Testes

How do the sperm cells get to the penis from the testes? Is there a direct route between the two?

No, the communication between the testes and the penis is quite indirect, and the course from one to the other is rather long and tortuous. We can get a clearer understanding of this pathway by looking at the diagram of the male organs. The testes are made up of a very large number of fine hairlike tubules in which the sperm are formed.

The Epididymis

These tubules gradually join together and then emerge at the top of the testes and connect with a special organ which carries the long name of epididymis, and in which the sperm undergo a gradual maturing process. It lies alongside the testes, to which it is closely attached, and consists of a very much coiled and convoluted duct. While the epididymis is only about two inches long and a quarter of an inch wide, the tube of which it is made up is very extensive. It has been calculated that if this duct were unwound and stretched lengthwise it would extend for some twenty feet.

Do you mean that a tube twenty feet long is compressed in so small a space?

Yes, and it is an example of some of the remarkable complexities in the structure of the body. The width of this tube is extremely small; it is only about one sixtieth of an inch in diameter, which would correspond to the size of a coarse cotton thread. At its lower end the epididymis is joined to and empties into a larger tube or duct, called the sperm duct or vas deferens.

The Vas Deferens

The vas deferens, usually called simply the vas, curves upward in the scrotum, passes through a canal in the groin and enters the lower part of the abdomen, or pelvis. Here it turns down again, and finally opens into the back part of the urethra. Its length is about sixteen inches and its diameter about one eighth of an inch. The walls of the vas are fairly thick, so that it can be felt easily in the scrotum as it passes up into the groin.

Do all the sperm cells have to travel this rather roundabout way?

Yes, indeed. And if for any reason this path is obstructed either in the epididymis or in the vas, the spermatozoa from that particular side will be unable to pass through. If it happens on both sides, the man will be sterile.

How can these canals become blocked?

Usually through injury or disease. A rather frequent cause is a gonorrheal inflammation. If the inflammation happens to be bilateral —that is, if it occurs on both sides—it is very apt to result in a blockage of both ducts and lead to sterility.

Would there be no seminal discharge at all then?

No, the seminal discharge would still continue. As I mentioned before, the bulk of fluid which is ejaculated comes from the other accessory sex glands—the seminal vesicles and the prostate; these are not affected by the blocking of the vas.

The Seminal Vesicles

What is the function of these other sex glands?

The seminal vesicles—there are two of them—are saclike organs which lie at the base of the bladder, and are connected through a special duct with the vas deferens. They produce a gelatinous, yellowish secretion of their own which mixes with the sperm, thickens the seminal fluid and gives it greater volume. This secretion also contains a special sugar, called fructose, which provides the sperm cells with the energy required for their vitality.

The Prostate

The prostate is another gland which takes part in the reproductive process. It is located around the urethra, right below the bladder and in front of the rectum. During the ejaculation, the prostate contracts and adds its own thin, milky secretion, which is alkaline in character, to the seminal fluid. The function of this secretion is not clearly understood as yet, but it is believed that, among other things, it contains a ferment which helps to liquefy the gelatinous semen after it is ejaculated.

What connection, Doctor, does the prostate have with the urinary organs? I understand that prostate trouble is often accompanied by urinary disturbances.

That is so. The prostate, while primarily a sex organ, lies in the very path of the urinary outlet, so that disorders of this gland are apt to give rise both to sexual and to urinary symptoms. Because of its location and function it is subject to disturbances from both these sources. A rather frequent cause of prostatic disease is the extension of an unchecked gonorrheal infection. This infection is usually limited to the lower or front part of the urethra, but it may pass upward and involve the prostate. Prostatic infections, however, may be caused by other organisms as well.

A relative of mine had some urinary trouble not long ago and his case was diagnosed as an enlargement of the prostate. Recently he was operated upon, and the prostate, I understand, was removed. What causes the prostate to enlarge?

The reasons for the enlargement of the prostate are not clearly understood as yet, but it is accepted now that it is not due to any venereal or other infection. The prostate has a general tendency to grow larger after middle age, that is after about the age of fifty, and in some people this increase in size may become quite pronounced in later life. Because of its anatomical position around the base of the bladder and the urethra, this enlargement may cause an obstruction to the passage of urine and lead to difficulty and frequency of urination and other distressing symptoms and constitutional disturbances. In advanced cases it sometimes becomes necessary to remove a part of or the entire prostate in order to alleviate the condition.

What effect does prostate trouble have on reproduction?

Probably very little. If the prostate is badly infected, its secretion may possibly decrease the vitality of the sperm, but usually prostatic infections do not affect reproductive capacity.

If the prostate gland has been removed, however, there will be little or no seminal fluid discharged, because of the resulting anatomical changes. The sexual capacity is not much disturbed, but because of the absence of the seminal discharge the man is, of course, likely to become infertile. As a rule, though, such operations are performed on men of fairly advanced age when the question of reproduction is no longer a factor.

The Penis

If the semen is made up of several different secretions, where do they mix together?

They are all brought together in the back part of the urethra, the channel which runs through the penis, and are discharged during the ejaculation. The penis is the male copulatory organ and serves primarily to bring the seminal fluid into the female genital tract. By its roots it is firmly attached to the bony parts of the pelvis. The external or visible part consists of a body, or shaft, and a head, or glans, at the tip of which is the opening of the urethra. The entire organ is covered with a rather loose, thin and elastic skin which extends as a double fold over the glans. The projecting portion of the skin is called the prepuce, or foreskin, and is the part which is removed when a circumcision is performed. The surface of the penis, and particularly of the glans, is richly supplied with nerve endings and is very sensitive to touch.

The Erection

Ordinarily the penis is flaccid and limp and hangs down rather loosely in front of the scrotum. In this condition the foreskin almost completely covers the glans. During sexual excitation and the process of erection the penis changes in size and direction; it becomes rigid, tense, enlarged and elevated. The foreskin is retracted so that the head, or glans, becomes partly or entirely exposed. This change is made possible by the peculiar spongelike structure of the organ. All through the penis there are a large number of small spaces. When these spaces are empty and their walls collapsed, the organ is flaccid; when they become distended with an increased inflow of blood, the penis becomes firm and erect. Its blood vessels, the arteries and the veins, are so constructed that they can allow an increased inflow and a diminished outflow of blood at the same time, so that all the spaces become engorged and distended. In addition there is a great deal of elastic tissue in the penis which permits a considerable change in the dimensions of the organ. During an erection, it becomes both longer and wider.

What is considered the normal size of the penis?

The average length of the nonerect penis, measuring from the back to the tip, is about three and three-quarters inches, and its circumference around the shaft is approximately three and a quarter inches. During an erection, the length increases on an average to five and a half or six inches and the circumference to about four and a half or five inches. These measurements are, however, only approximate, for the size of the organ is subject to marked individual variations.

Do the dimensions of the organ depend upon the general physique of the man?

Not particularly. The dimensions of the penis seem to be controlled by factors other than those which determine the general build of the body, perhaps by the internal secretions of the sex glands. Measurements of the organ in a large number of men have been taken, and no definite correlation between the size of the body and that of the penis has been found.

Has the size of the penis any relation to the man's sexual power?

Not to any degree. There is apparently little relation between the size of the penis and sexual capacity. I have seen many men who were sexually very active in spite of a comparatively small-sized organ, and also many men who had a low degree of potency although their penile dimensions were far above the average.

Circumcision

How about circumcision, Doctor? Is it of any particular value for a man to be circumcised?

Circumcision, as I mentioned, consists in the removal of the foreskin which covers the greater part of the head of the penis. It is probably one of the oldest surgical operations and has been practiced since prehistoric times by peoples in different parts of the world. How it originated is not definitely known. Some maintain that the removal of the foreskin was in the nature of a sacrificial offering which was gradually substituted for more deforming and incapacitating practices of this type. Others claim that it originated as a tribal custom and was regarded as a tribal badge, or else that it was an initiation ceremony and a preparation for the marital act, although among some peoples the practice was later transferred to early infancy. It may also have arisen as a hygienic practice which gradually assumed the character of a religious rite.

Under the foreskin there is usually an accumulation of a whitish, pasty material, called smegma, which has to be cleansed away at frequent intervals to avoid local irritation and inflammation. The removal of the foreskin exposes the parts and permits greater cleanliness of the organ. Hence it is often recommended as a desirable hygienic measure.

Would you advise circumcision as a routine practice?

Not necessarily. If the foreskin happens to be especially long or so tight that it cannot be easily drawn back, circumcision is advisable. Ordinarily, however, there is no special need for it. As far as we know there seems to be no difference either in the degree of sexual desire or in sexual capacity between circumcised and uncircumcised men.

Precoital Secretion

During an erection a little bit of fluid sometimes appears at the tip of the penis. Is this a part of the semen?

No, this fluid is not a part of the ejaculation. You will recall that the urethra, the canal which runs through the penis, serves a double purpose: it is the passage through which both the urine and the seminal fluid come out. Now, urine is generally acid in character, and acids have a harmful effect upon the sperm. To counteract any possible ill effect from this source, certain glands along the urethra pour out an alkaline secretion into this canal during sexual excitement. This presumably neutralizes any acids which may remain in the urethra, so that the seminal fluid will not be harmed during its passage. This secretion may appear at the opening of the penis, or meatus, as a drop of sticky moisture. Some believe that this fluid may also serve to lubricate the urethra for the passage of the seminal fluid.

Does this secretion contain any sperm cells?

Not as a rule. Ordinarily this fluid appears as a colorless, transparent, somewhat sticky secretion and is free from any sperm. Under certain circumstances, however, it is possible for a slight leakage of the seminal fluid to take place during sexual excitement even before the actual ejaculation. This too will appear as a slight discharge at the meatus. In a special study of this particular question, I found that in a small percentage of cases this discharge did contain spermatozoa. Their presence can be determined by a microscopic examination of this precoital secretion.

The Ejaculation

Is the seminal fluid being formed at all times, or only at the time of sexual stimulation?

The various secretions which go to make up the seminal fluid are being produced continuously, but the actual blending of these fluids into semen occurs only at the moment of ejaculation. It is at this time that muscular contractions of the genital tract force the sperm from the vas, together with the secretions of the seminal vesicles, into the urinary canal. At the same time the contractions of the prostate force its own fluid out through a number of small openings into the urinary canal close to the place where the sperm fluid enters. There all the secretions are mixed together and are ejaculated in several spurts through the penis.

If the seminal fluid and the urine pass through the same canal, how is it that the two do not mix during the ejaculation?

This involves a rather interesting point. The two do not mix because of a fine adaptation of the nervous and muscular mechanism of the urinary and genital systems. When an erection takes place, the opening between the bladder and the urethra is automatically shut off by a reflex contraction of the appropriate muscles, thus keeping the urine from passing into the urethra during this process and ejaculation. It is another illustration of the delicate adjustments which we find so often in the human body.

The Sperm

About how many sperm cells are present in one ejaculation?

An amazing number indeed. In the average ejaculation, which consists of nearly a teaspoonful of fluid, there are some two to five hundred million sperm. When it comes to the question of the propagation of the race, nature appears to have been extremely liberal in the supply of male reproductive material.

Most of the sperm, incidentally, are concentrated in the first part of the ejaculate. Thus, if a man should discharge his fluid in two successive portions at the time of the ejaculation, the greatest number of sperm cells would be found in the first part. This is of interest in connection with the problems of fertility and sterility in marriage.

When the seminal fluid is first ejaculated, it is gelatinous in character, but within three to fifteen minutes it becomes liquefied. In this freshly ejaculated gelatinous semen the sperm are found motionless or almost motionless, but as liquefaction takes place, they begin to move more and more actively.

The sperm must be very small indeed if several hundred million are gathered in less than a teaspoonful of fluid.

Yes, each sperm measures only about one six-hundredths of an inch in length. With an ordinary microscope, however, they can be seen very clearly. It is a very interesting sight indeed to look at a drop of seminal fluid under the microscope. In a fresh specimen every drop swarms with actively moving sperm. It has been calculated that the sperm can travel about one eighth of an inch in a minute, or, in other words, an inch in approximately eight minutes.

What does a sperm cell look like?

A sperm resembles a minute elongated tadpole. It has a rounded head, a small middle piece and a long, slender tail. The head and middle piece contain the important elements which take part in reproduction and heredity. It is here that the chromosomes and genes of which we spoke last time are located. The tail lashes rapidly from side to side and causes the movement of the cell, although the mechanism of the motion seems to reside in the middle piece. After a time the movements become slower and slower, until they cease altogether; the sperm remains immobile and soon dies.

How long can the sperm remain alive after the ejaculation?

That depends upon the environment in which they are placed after emission. I shall discuss with you later the life of the sperm in the genital tract of the female. Outside the body, their length of life depends largely upon the temperature at which they are kept. Under ordinary room temperature, sperm may remain alive for twenty-four hours and longer after ejaculation. In a warm temperature, their motility is speeded up so that their energy is quickly spent and their life span shortened. If placed in a refrigerator, however, they can be kept alive for several days. The cold temperature inactivates them temporarily, and when they are later warmed their activity reappears. If frozen instantaneously, the sperm can be kept in a dormant state for months and perhaps years, and then revived at will.

Are the sperm being produced in the testes continuously?

Well, in many of the lower animals the production of sperm is seasonal, and is limited to only a few months of the year; during the remaining months, the testes are inactive as far as sperm production is concerned. In most higher animals, however, the sperm are generated all through the year. Man belongs to this latter group, and his sperm production is presumably continuous.

Suppose a man had one ejaculation and then an hour later, let us say, he had another. Would this second discharge contain as many sperm as the first?

Probably not, though this will depend upon the degree to which the vasa deferentia empty their contents during the first emission. A second ejaculation soon after the first is likely to contain less fluid and fewer sperm. It may take some time, perhaps twenty-four hours, for the reservoirs to fill up to their normal capacity after a complete emptying. If ejaculations follow in rapid succession, the fluid discharged later will be very thin and will contain fewer cells.

If a man refrains from sexual relations and has few semen discharges, does the retained semen have any beneficial effect?

This is a question about which there has been a great deal of discussion. In the Oneida Community, an American group which was organized during the middle of the last century, the men consciously abstained from discharging their seminal fluid during intercourse partly as a contraceptive measure and partly in the belief that this practice would benefit their health and increase their vigor. They called this form of sexual union "male continence." Whether it proved to be of any particular value to their health was not, however, properly studied.

As a matter of fact, according to the data reported by Kinsey, early and frequent sex activity does not apparently impair sex function and capacity later in life.

What happens to the sperm if no ejaculation takes place?

The sperm present in the vas gradually die and are broken down and absorbed by the white and other blood cells of the body. In animals isolated from sexual contact, degenerated masses of sperm are found in the seminal ducts and passages. It has also been shown that the first ejaculation after a long period of abstinence contains less active or vigorous sperm than those which appear in ejaculations after moderately frequent intercourse, indicating that the sperm tend to lose their vitality if they remain in the body for a long time.

Is there any relation, Doctor, between the male sex hormones and the seminal fluid?

The only relation is that sperm cells and hormones both are produced in the testes. The two, however, are formed by different parts of the gland.

Hormones

What exactly is a hormone, Doctor?

The term "hormone" is applied to chemical substances which are produced by certain glands and are carried by the blood to various organs of the body whose functions they influence. Because these secretions are not emptied through any ducts or channels but enter directly into the blood, hormones are also called internal secretions. There are several hormone-producing glands located in various parts of the body. The more important ones are the pituitary at the base of the brain, the thyroid in the neck, the adrenals near the kidneys, and the sex glands—that is, the testes and the ovaries, sometimes also called gonads. Most of the hormones, as a matter of fact, play an important role in sex and reproduction, and we shall refer to them at various times as we go along.

Hormones have the power of initiating and stimulating the activities of different organs and tissues. It is believed that each hormone has a specific role in the mechanism of the body. The various glands, however, have a reciprocal action upon each other, and if one does not function properly the others too may become affected.

Does the semen contain any special hormone, Doctor?

As far as we know, not in an amount that can be of any importance. As I mentioned, the testes produce the sperm and the male sex hormones, but the two are formed by different parts of the testes. The sperm pass into the seminal ducts, while the hormones are absorbed directly into the bloodstream and are carried throughout the body.

Primary and Secondary Sexual Characters

What is the special function of the sex hormones?

As far as the male sex hormone is concerned, its specific function is to control the development of the so-called secondary male sexual characteristics, the qualities which distinguish the male from the female. There are certain features, as you know, both structural and functional, which are found in one sex and not in the other, and which differentiate the male from the female. The sex organs themselves constitute the primary sexual characters. When a child is born, one tells its sex by looking at the genitals. As it grows older, however, other characteristics appear which serve to differentiate the sexes. At puberty, the boy develops a growth of hair on his face, his larynx enlarges so that his voice becomes deeper, and the build of his body becomes distinctly masculine. The girl gradually develops a more rounded contour, fuller breasts, broader hips, and a feminine hair distribution. These are called the secondary sexual characters. They are present in many animal species, too. The rooster, for example, grows a comb and spurs, the stag develops antlers, rams grow horns, and the plumage of many birds varies with their sex; all these are secondary sexual characteristics.

Castration

Then the differences between a man and a woman are controlled largely by their sex hormones?

Yes, to a great degree. If the testes of an animal are removed soon after its birth, that animal will not develop the features or traits of his sex. The castrated cock, for instance, does not grow a comb and wattles, he does not crow, he lacks pugnacity and pays no attention to the females of his species. In the stag and in the ram this operation prevents the development of antlers and horns. The differences between the bull and the steer, the stallion and the gelding are due primarily to the effects of the removal of the sex glands. Such operations have been performed from the earliest times on horses, bulls, dogs, cats and other domestic animals for experimental or, more usually, for economic purposes. Castrated animals are more docile, more easily managed, and they tend to lose their sexual desire and drive.

What happens if the sex glands are removed in man?

The removal of the glands in a boy before puberty markedly influences his later development, appearance and personality. This operation has not infrequently been performed on boys for a number of different reasons. In Oriental countries, for instance, it has been done in order to produce an unsexed type of individual, or eunuch, to serve as an attendant in harems. In Italy, castration of boys was a common practice at one time for the purpose of providing sopranos for church choirs. Magnus Hirschfeld, who has made many studies of sex practices, states that during the Middle Ages one could see signs in the windows of most barbers and male nurses in Rome reading: "Here castrations are done cheaply." Among a certain religious group of Russia, known as the Skoptzi, the removal of the sex organs was practiced as a part of their rituals. Thus a considerable amount of information concerning the effects of castration in the male has been accumulated. In general it has been found that a boy deprived of his testes does not develop the masculine secondary sexual characters, and tends to resemble more a neuter type of individual. His face remains beardless, his larynx does not enlarge and he retains a high-pitched, soprano voice. He also tends to deposit an excess of fat. His sexual organs remain undeveloped and his sexual impulses never fully awaken.

What happens if a man's glands are removed later in life?

The changes that follow castration after puberty are much less marked. Once the secondary sexual characteristics have appeared, they do not recede completely after castration, although various changes in growth, in fat deposit, in psychological and emotional attitudes do take place. Sexual desire and sexual potency may be retained for a long time after the operation, but in some cases they are greatly diminished or even entirely lost.

Gland Transplantation

Incidentally, some very interesting work has been done with gland transplantation. It has been found possible to remove the glands from one animal and transplant them into another of the same or of a different species. Frequently these transplants "take" and continue to grow in the body of the host. Such transplantations were first performed for experimental purposes in the middle of the last century, and they have been continued on a wider scale in more recent years. Eugen Steinach, working with rats and guinea pigs, found that if a young animal was deprived of his testes, it was possible to cause the development of his secondary male sexual characteristics by implanting in him a testis from another animal. Later he went even a step further: he removed the sex glands from female animals and substituted for them the testis of a male, and he reported that the females became masculinized—they increased in size, their genital organs changed somewhat to the male type, and they adopted a male sexual behavior toward the females. Similar results have been obtained with birds. Female birds in whom a male gland was implanted developed the comb and wattles, the spurs, the plumage and even the sexual behavior of the males.

Have gland transplantations ever been performed on men?

Yes, they have. One of the first to transplant a testis was the American surgeon Lydston. In 1914 he obtained the testicle of a man who had committed suicide, and transplanted it into his own scrotum in order to observe the effects. He claimed then that the operation benefited him greatly, improving his health and increasing his vigor. Similar operations were later performed by other investigators. Voronoff employed the testes of simians—the famous "monkey glands"—for the purpose, and he gave a glowing account of the results. These benefits were actually the result of the psychic stimulation of the individual.

Testicular Extracts; the Male Hormone

I understand that male sex hormones are now frequently prescribed by physicians. Are they of any value?

The use of extracts from the male glands for the purpose of bringing about physical and sexual rejuvenation dates back to the famous physiologist Brown-Séquard. At the age of seventy-one Brown-Séquard injected himself with extracts from the testicles of a dog, and in 1889 he made an enthusiastic report of the results. He claimed that his general health, his muscular power and his mental activity were amazingly stimulated. He felt, he said, like a youth with all the youth's vigor. Since then testicular extracts have been employed very widely, but Brown-Séquard's claims have not been substantiated. There is little evidence that any beneficial effects were obtained from the testicular gland extracts formerly available.

However, more concentrated and purified extract of the male hormone has been produced. This has been obtained from the testes, from the urine of males, and from other sources. The male hormone has also been isolated in pure form and produced synthetically from various chemical substances. This product, known as testosterone, has been reported to induce the development of the male secondary sexual characteristics in animals whose testes had previously been removed. In female animals it is apt to produce physical changes typical of the male. If testosterone is injected into a hen, for example, she will develop a pronounced growth of the comb and actually begin to crow like a rooster; if it is administered to a female canary, she will begin to sing like a male. The hormone has, therefore, a masculinizing effect.

Clinically, testosterone has in some instances shown favorable effects on men suffering from certain kinds of sexual deficiencies. It has been recommended for use in older men as a general stimulant, as well as for the restoration of waning sexual potency. The process of aging, however, involves not merely the genital system but the entire organism, and it is questionable whether the injection of any hormones can arrest or reverse these general systemic changes. Besides, men and women are subject to so many psychic and emotional influences that it is often very difficult to evaluate the results of therapeutic measures of this sort.

We have covered many phases of the sexual physiology of the male today, and we still have to consider the female reproductive organs. Shall we leave that for tomorrow?

CHAPTER III

THE BIOLOGY
OF MARRIAGE
THE FEMALE SEX ORGANS

We are to continue today with our discussion of sexual anatomy and physiology, and I will start with a description of the female reproductive system.

The Role of the Female in Reproduction

The role of the female in reproduction is very much more complicated than that of the male. In the begetting of offspring, as we have seen, the male's part consists merely in the production of sperm and their transmission to the female. With the deposit of his sperm, his role, as far as the physiological processes of procreation are concerned, is completed. The female, too, has to produce her sex cells, the eggs, but, in addition, it is within her body that the manifold steps of the development and growth of the embryo take place. It is within her that the male and female sex cells meet and unite; it is in her body that the fertilized egg nests and develops into its mature form; and it is with her secretions that she nourishes the newborn during the early period of its life.

All the processes of childbearing go on within the body of the woman. Her reproductive organs and functions are, therefore, considerably more diversified and complicated than those of the male. In fact, they play a greater role in her general biological activities.

In the male, as we have seen, the sex organs, which in the main lie outside his body, include, first, the glands which are concerned with the production of the sperm and the seminal fluid, and, second, the passages and organs which serve to carry the fluid and to convey it into the female. In the female, similarly, there are, first, the sex glands which produce the female sex cells or eggs, and, second, the tubes and canals for the passage of the egg cells and the reception of the sperm. In addition, however, there are also the organs which are concerned with the development and nutrition of the embryo. All these structures are located inside the body of the woman and are known as the internal sex organs. The external genitals are not directly concerned in the process of reproduction, and I shall speak of them separately later.

The Female Pelvis

Our knowledge of female anatomy is very vague indeed. Can you show us a diagram of the organs?

Yes, this diagram (Figure 2, page 65) may make the female reproductive system clearer to you. It represents a side view of the pelvis, similar to the diagram of the male pelvis which we saw last time, and it shows the several organs which lie in this region between the lower part of the spine in the back and the abdominal wall in the front. I shall point them out first, and we can then discuss each one more fully. Here is the rectum close to the spinal column, and here is the bladder, near the abdominal wall in front, just as in the male. Between the two you will notice another canal or passage, the vagina. Projecting into the vagina from above is a pear-shaped body, the uterus, or womb. Extending from the uterus on each side are two narrow ducts, the tubes, and at the outer end of each tube is a small glandular body, the ovary.

Are the ovaries the sex glands of the woman?

Yes, the ovaries are the female sex glands and correspond to the testes of the male. Other glands, especially the pituitary at the base of the brain, also play a very important role in the sex physiology of the woman, but the term "sex glands" refers to the ovaries. These are located inside the body, in the lower part of the abdomen. Each ovary is oval in form, about an inch and a half long, an inch wide, and half an inch thick, and can be compared in size and shape to a large unshelled almond. The primary function of the ovaries is to develop the female germ cells which are called ova, or eggs, but, like the testes, the ovaries also produce internal secretions, or hormones, which greatly influence many of the woman's bodily functions.

At birth each ovary contains many thousands of potential egg cells. They are potential because they are only in a very immature and primitive state at this time, and they still have to undergo a very complicated process of growth and development before they become fully ripened. As a matter of fact, very few of the eggs ever reach the complete state of development. Out of the thousands of primitive eggs, only a few hundred at most ever become fully mature human ova.

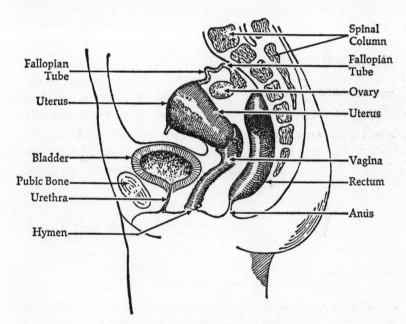

FIGURE 2. *Female Genital Organs (side view)*

Ovulation

Do the eggs develop within the ovary?

Yes. The ripening process goes on in the ovary and begins with the onset of puberty. It is from this time on that the primitive eggs commence to develop and mature at periodic intervals. About every twenty-eight days several of these cells increase in size and undergo a series of very complex changes. One of the eggs enlarges more than the others and becomes surrounded by a little sac of fluid, called a Graafian follicle, after the Dutch anatomist de Graaf, who, in 1672, first described these follicles. When fully developed, the follicle may reach a size of about half an inch in diameter. As it enlarges, it gradually makes its way to the surface of the ovary, where it looks and feels like a small blister. After a while the wall of the sac breaks, and the ripe egg, or ovum, is released from the gland. This process of the discharge of the mature ovum from the ovary is technically called ovulation.

After ovulation has taken place, the follicle fills up with new cells which form a new transitory gland within the ovary, which is yellowish in color and is called the "yellow body," or corpus luteum. A hormone which plays an important role in reproduction is produced by this newly formed body.

Since there is only one egg discharged each month, how is this function divided between the two ovaries? Is there any regular sequence?

It was formerly assumed that they functioned alternately—that is, that an egg matured in one ovary one month and in the other ovary the following month. It is now believed that such periodicity and rotation do not necessarily exist. Sometimes one ovary may function for several months in succession before an egg will begin to mature in the other.

What happens, Doctor, if one ovary is removed?

Well, if one ovary is removed, the other will entirely compensate for the loss. The remaining ovary will continue to produce an ovum every month, so that the reproductive capacity of the woman is not affected.

Does the release of the eggs from the ovaries take place during sexual relations like the discharge of the male sperm?

No, at least not so far as the human female is concerned. In certain animals, such as the rabbit or the cat, for instance, the release of the egg does depend upon the stimulus of the sexual relation, and occurs only after mating. In the woman, however, the cells mature and come out of the ovary entirely irrespective of sexual contact. It is possible that when an egg is fully ripened and ready to be released, the act of intercourse might hasten the process and bring about ovulation, but this is still a debatable point.

Furthermore, the manner of development and release of the germ cells differs greatly in the male and the female. The sperm presumably mature continuously in the testes and are discharged in large numbers during each ejaculation. The eggs, on the other hand, ripen only periodically, and they are released from the ovaries only one at a time at regular monthly intervals. This release has no relation to sexual contact.

Compared to the lavishness in the production of sperm, the formation of eggs seems to be rather meager, doesn't it?

Yes, the difference is striking. Under ordinary circumstances only one egg is released every twenty-eight days, and the number of eggs which may develop during a year would be only about twelve or thirteen. As a woman's reproductive life lasts approximately thirty years, the total number of her matured eggs would range between three and four hundred. This is in marked contrast to the male, whose every ejaculation contains millions of sperm.

Ovulation and Menstruation

Is there any relation, Doctor, between the discharge of the egg cell and the menstrual flow of the woman?

Yes, indeed. There is a very close physiological connection between the two processes. It is very generally accepted now that the structural and functional changes which lead to the appearance of the menstrual flow are dependent to a large extent upon the activities of the ovary. Certain chemical substances, or hormones, which are produced in the follicle of the ripening egg before, during and after the discharge of the ovum, are the agents which initiate the physiological processes of menstruation.

Does a woman menstruate at the time that an egg is being discharged?

No, the two phenomena are not simultaneous. For a long time there was a considerable divergence of medical opinion as to when during the menstrual month ovulation took place. Ovulation generally occurs about midway between two periods, and it is the release of the egg from the ovary and the subsequent changes in the follicle which really initiate the next menstrual cycle. In other words, menstruation occurs about twelve to sixteen days following ovulation. I might mention, however, that under certain circumstances menses may occur without ovulation as well as ovulation without menstruation.

Can a woman tell when an egg has ripened and is being discharged from the ovary? Does she feel anything at the time?

Not as a rule. Some women can have a cramplike feeling in the lower part of the abdomen or a slight bloodstaining during the middle of the menstrual month, and it is possible that this corresponds to the time when the egg is being expelled from the ovary. Ordinarily, however, a woman is not at all aware of the process and cannot tell when ovulation occurs.

The Egg Cell (Ovum)

What does a human egg look like? How does it compare with a sperm cell?

The egg cell is quite different from a sperm in structure and in form. It is spheroidal or rounded in shape, has no power of locomotion, and is stationary and passive. It is much larger than a sperm, about one two-hundredths of an inch in diameter, and just visible to the naked eye. Even so, however, it is extremely small—less than the size of an ordinary period on a printed page. The outside of the egg is surrounded by a jellylike wall or shell, and the inside is filled with a large number of minute fat droplets, referred to as yolk matter. In the center of the cell, or somewhat to one side of it, lies the nucleus which holds the chromosomes with their genes, the carriers of the maternal hereditary qualities.

Does a human egg also contain yolk? Is it anything like a hen's egg?

In its essential structure the human egg is quite analogous to a bird's egg, except that it is, of course, much smaller and is not surrounded by a hard shell. The difference in size, however, is due primarily to a difference in the quantity of stored nutritive material. The fertilized egg of the hen does not remain in the body of the female, but is passed out to be incubated outside. The development of the chick goes on within the egg quite independently of the mother, and hence the egg must possess a large quantity of food material to supply the growing embryo until it is ready to hatch. It also needs a shell for protection. In the human species, the method of development is quite different. After fertilization—that is, after the union of the egg with a sperm—the embryo remains in the body of the mother and for many months continues to obtain its nourishment directly from her. There is no need, therefore, for storing up much food material in the egg itself, and its size is consequently small.

The Fallopian Tubes

What happens to the ripe egg after it comes out of the ovary?

If you will look at the diagram you will notice a narrow tube or duct extending from the ovary to the womb, or uterus. There are two tubes, one on each side, and they are known as the Fallopian tubes, after the anatomist Fallopius, who first described them. Each tube is about five inches long, with a very narrow canal running through it. Near the ovary, the end of the tube is somewhat expanded and has fringelike projections which come up close to the gland at the time of ovulation. As the egg is extruded from the ovary, it is drawn into or caught up by the tube. Here it slowly makes its way inward until it finally reaches the uterus.

I thought you said that the egg could not move by itself. How does it get to the uterus?

You are quite right. The egg is entirely immobile. It is moved forward in the tube partly by the muscular contractions of the tube itself which force it onward, and partly by the aid of very fine hairlike projections which line the tubal canal. These projections, known as cilia, constantly wave in an inward direction, and their motion aids in propelling the egg toward the uterus. It usually takes from three to four days for the egg to be transported through the tube to the uterus.

The Uterus

Do I understand correctly, Doctor, that the words "womb" and "uterus" apply to the same organ?

Yes, the terms "womb" and "uterus" are synonymous. "Uterus" is the medical term. In size and shape the uterus appears somewhat like a flattened pear. Its wider part, the body, is at the top and its narrower part, the neck, or cervix, at the bottom. The average size of the uterus is from two and a half to three and a half inches in length and from two to two and a half inches in width, being larger in a woman who has borne children. Its walls are very thick and made up largely of muscle. In the center of the uterus is a cavity with three openings leading from it, two on top which communicate with the Fallopian tubes on each side, and one at the bottom which opens into the vagina (Figure 3, below). The cavity is lined with a special membrane which is very richly supplied with blood and which undergoes many complex structural changes every month, as a part of the process of menstruation. It is into this cavity that the egg enters from the tube.

How long does the egg remain in the uterus?

Well, it may stay there for a few days or for many months, depending upon whether during its journey through the tube it was fertilized by a sperm. An unfertilized egg soon either disintegrates and is absorbed or may possibly pass out through the lower opening of the uterus into the vagina and from there to the outside.

A fertilized egg, however, attaches itself to the wall of the uterus, and nests there for about nine months. During this period it slowly undergoes a series of remarkable transformations and differentiations until it emerges as the newborn baby. The uterus serves as an incubator and feeding place for the fetus. It is a place in which the embryo finds not only protection and warmth but also its necessary

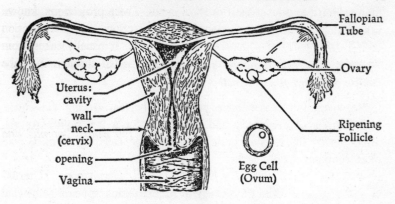

FIGURE 3. *Internal Female Genital Organs (front view)*

nourishment. The egg, as we saw, contains a small quantity of nutritive material which carries it through the initial stages of its growth. Then, however, it must obtain nourishment from some other source. This it gets, as we shall see later, from the mother's body through a special apparatus which develops at the site of its attachment to the uterus. At the end of the period of pregnancy, when the baby is ready to be delivered, the strong muscular walls of the uterus contract and force the child out of the mother's body.

If an egg is not fertilized, does the woman know when it is coming out of her body?

No. The passage of the egg is not accompanied by any sensation, and the woman is not aware of its occurrence. In fact, the egg most likely disintegrates completely before it comes out. It is so small that it can hardly be seen with the naked eye, and, as far as I know, it has never been found in the discharges from the vagina.

The fact that the ovaries of women form eggs was demonstrated more than a hundred years ago by von Baer. But ripe human ova had never been seen until 1928, when Allen and his co-workers, after an extensive and intensive search, succeeded in finding and observing several human egg cells in the tubes. In three instances, single cells were found, and in one case a pair of twin eggs, making a total of five eggs. Incidentally, you may find a fascinating account of the long search for the solution to the mysteries of human reproduction in Guttmacher's book *Life in the Making*.

When an egg is fertilized and pregnancy occurs, does the ovary continue to form other egg cells?

No, ovulation ceases once pregnancy begins. During the entire nine months of pregnancy and sometimes for a few months thereafter, during the nursing period, no new egg cells are formed, and menstruation does not occur.

The Physiology of Menstruation

What, Doctor, is the function of menstruation?

Every mature egg as it is released from the ovary is a potential embryo. If fertilized by a sperm it will develop into a new life. This development, as we just saw, goes on largely in the uterus, the lining of which has to undergo certain changes in order to accommodate the fertilized egg. Every time an egg matures, hormones are sent to the uterus which initiate structural changes in its lining and prepare it for the coming of the egg. The lining receives an increased blood supply and becomes swollen and thickened. If the egg is fertilized, this thickened wall continues to grow and forms a nesting place for the embryo. If, however, the egg has not been fertilized, there is no need for this newly formed tissue and, through the action of other hormones, it is broken down and shed from the body. Together with an accompanying discharge of blood and mucus from the uterus, this constitutes the menstrual flow. In other words, menstruation is usually indicative of the fact that a mature egg cell has not been fertilized.

At what age is it normal for a girl to begin to menstruate?

Menstruation begins, on an average, between the thirteenth and fourteenth years, but there are wide variations, and the first menstrual period may occur at any time between the ninth and seventeenth years. These variations may be due to any of a number of factors—to climate, race, heredity, diet, glandular conditions and even psychological factors.

How regular should a woman's periods be?

The average interval from the first day of one menstrual period to the onset of the next is about twenty-eight days, but few women are altogether regular in their cycles. Variations of several days are quite frequent, and cycles ranging from twenty-five to thirty-five days are noted by a large number of women who keep an accurate record of their periods. Many factors, both physical and emotional, affect the regularity of the cycle.

Does a woman lose much blood at each menstruation?

The average quantity of blood lost during the days of the flow is about two to four ounces, or approximately half a cupful. It comes out from the uterus not as a steady flow but in irregular spurts, squeezed out by the contractions of the uterine muscles. The menstrual blood is unusual in that it does not clot readily.

Painful Menstruation

Why is menstruation sometimes so painful, Doctor? I know women who have such severe cramps that they have to go to bed for the first day of the period.

Under normal conditions a woman usually should have no pain during menstruation. It is a fact, nevertheless, that not many women are entirely free from any unpleasant sensations at this time. The discomfort may vary from a slight feeling of heaviness in the pelvic region, and perhaps a general indisposition and irritability, to quite severe abdominal cramps, backache, intestinal disturbances and marked depression. The causes of these manifestations are not yet clearly understood in all instances. Underdevelopment of the genital organs, displacements of the uterus, inflammatory conditions in the pelvic region, unbalanced hormone production, general debility, marked constipation, and many other factors may cause painful menses. Psychiatrists often ascribe menstrual discomforts to emotional disturbances. To some degree, the present widespread prevalence of painful menstruation may be due to our accelerated mode of life, to faulty dietary habits, to lack of adequate muscular development, to neurotic tendencies and similar factors. The menstrual phenomenon is still often regarded with traditional taboos, and even women themselves tend to view this process as a feminine affliction rather than as a normal physiological function. Such an attitude often leads to an emotional state which contributes considerably to the pain and discomfort. Just as there is no one cause for painful menstuation or dysmenorrhea, there is also no one specific treatment. There are, however, many effective methods that may be tried on an individual basis.

If a girl suffers painful menstruation, is the pain likely to be diminished or relieved after marriage?

That would depend, of course, upon the underlying cause of the discomfort. It sometimes happens, it is true, that the physical and emotional changes brought about by the marriage relationship may indirectly influence menstrual function and menstrual pain, but this is not invariably the case. Quite frequently, however, a woman will be free from subsequent menstrual discomforts once she has gone through a pregnancy and childbirth, due to the local and systemic changes which accompany the processes of reproduction.

A pelvic condition known as endometriosis is sometimes the cause of severe menstrual pains. Some physicians maintain that this condition is associated with the postponement of childbearing, and that early and frequent pregnancies may prevent or cure it. But the facts have not as yet been definitely established.

Hygiene of Menstruation

Is bathing permissible during the menstrual period? I have heard many different opinions about it.

There seems to be no sufficient reason for the restrictions put upon the use of water and cleansing during the menses. On the contrary, cleanliness is particularly indicated at this time. It is advisable, in fact, to bathe and cleanse the external genitals thoroughly several times daily during the menstrual flow. Nor is there any objection to tub bathing, providing the water is kept at a comfortable temperature. Extremes of heat or cold are inadvisable, and that is why lake or sea swimming is not to be recommended except in Southern areas.

The most convenient form of bathing during the menstrual period is probably the shower or sponge bath.

What about athletic activities during menstruation? Are exercise and sports advisable at this time?

Moderate physical activity during the menstrual period is not harmful. A girl may engage in any form of activity to which she is usually accustomed, unless the flow happens to be profuse or the accompanying discomfort rather marked. Severe exertion, however, and particularly competitive sports, should be avoided in order not to cause undue bodily fatigue or any increased congestion of the pelvic organs.

Are there any objections to using tampons during menstruation?

Ordinarily the use of compressed absorbent cotton in the form of vaginal tampons is quite harmless. They may fail to provide adequate protection, especially during the days when the flow is heavy, but unless an inflammatory condition is present their use has no ill effect on the genital organs.

At what age does a woman stop menstruating altogether?

Menstruation usually ceases between the ages of forty-five and fifty. At this time the woman reaches her "change of life," or climacteric, technically known as the menopause. With the cessation of the menstrual cycles the childbearing period of a woman also comes to an end. The menopause is a natural transition in a woman's life and results primarily from a decrease in the functioning of the ovaries. The menopause does not appear suddenly; it is preceded by a period of one or more years during which the menstrual cycles and the quantity of the flow become increasingly irregular. This period in a woman's life is sometimes accompanied by a variety of symptoms, such as hot flashes, profuse perspiration, dizziness, headaches, insomnia, emotional instability and other nervous manifestations. Many of these symptoms, however, can now be alleviated by the use of various hormones.

The Vagina

Does the menstrual blood come only from the uterus? Does any of it come from the vagina?

The menstrual blood comes only from the uterus and none from the vagina. The vagina constitutes a path of communication between the uterus and the exterior. It is the receptive sex organ and genital passage of the woman, receiving the male organ and the seminal discharge during sexual contact, and carrying the menstrual flow and other uterine secretions to the outside. The vagina also serves as a channel for the passage of the newborn child on its way from the uterus, and hence it forms a part of the "birth canal."

As you see on the diagram (Figure 2, page 65) the vagina opens below to the outside. This opening is called the vaginal orifice, or mouth of the vagina, and in the virgin it is partially covered by a special membrane, called the hymen. Above, the vagina is closed all around, with the neck of the uterus indenting it and projecting into it. To the examining finger the neck feels like a small, firm knob in the center of which is a small depression, the opening into the cavity of the uterus. The walls of the vagina are pinkish in color and are thrown into numerous folds, so that the canal has a somewhat corrugated appearance.

Is there any possibility of an object being lost inside the body if it is introduced into the vagina?

No. Except for the opening to the outside, the vagina is closed all around, and its only communication with the inside of the body, the abdominal cavity, is through the tiny opening in the neck of the uterus. Ordinarily this orifice is very small, only about one fifth of an inch in diameter. A larger object cannot, therefore, pass through the vagina into the uterus, and certainly not into the inside of the body. There is no basis for the fear which some women have that tampons, for example, or other objects introduced into the vagina might "get lost" inside.

How wide is the opening to the vagina?

The vaginal orifice varies greatly in size. Before defloration—that is, before the hymen is dilated—the opening may measure about half an inch in diameter. In the married woman the diameter increases to one and a half and even two inches, depending upon the extent of her sexual experiences, the number of childbirths and other factors. The tissues around the orifice are very elastic so that during child-birth it can stretch to a width of more than four inches in order to permit the passage of the head of the newborn child. After delivery, however, the opening returns to nearly its previous size.

Does the size of the vagina itself vary in different women, Doctor?

In length the vaginal canal measures on an average from three to three and a half inches. This size, however, is subject to many in-dividual variations, as well as to changes which depend on the woman's sexual life and her reproductive history. The important fact, perhaps, is that the walls of the vagina are very elastic and the canal can be easily distended. Normally, the vaginal walls are prac-tically in apposition, touching each other, so that there is no actual vaginal cavity. When an object is introduced into the canal, however, the walls separate and are stretched apart. In other words, the vagina in the natural state may be compared to a collapsed balloon which ` can be dilated by the introduction of air, liquid, or a solid substance.

Does the vaginal canal change much in size after a woman has had sexual relations?

The sexual act in itself affects the size of the vaginal canal only to a slight degree. The variations in size depend largely upon natural anatomical differences, upon muscular tensions which result from emotional factors, and upon the extent of a woman's sexual experi-ence. I have seen unusually deep vaginas in virgins, and very shallow ones in women who had been married for many years. The changes in the depth and width of the canal after marriage are due largely to the enlargement and stretching which results from pregnancy and childbirth.

There is one thing that is not quite clear to me, Doctor. You said last time that during an erection the male organ may attain a size of about six inches. If the length of the vagina is only about three inches, isn't there a great disproportion between the male and female parts?

I expect to discuss with you later on the mechanism of coitus in some detail. As far as your question is concerned, however, I might point out now that the coital canal, or the path which the male organ takes during coitus, involves more than the mere length of the vagina. It includes also a certain part of the external genitals, which form what Dickinson, in his source book *Human Sex Anatomy,* calls the "funnel of entry" into the vagina. This funnel is about one and a half inches long. In addition, the tissues around the genitals as well as the vaginal walls themselves are distensible and compressible, so that in spite of the fact that the depth of the vagina is only a little over three inches, the total length of the coital passage of the female ordinarily averages from five and a half to six inches.

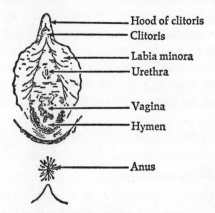

Hood of clitoris
Clitoris
Labia minora
Urethra
Vagina
Hymen
Anus

FIGURE 4. *External Female Genital Organs (front view)*

The External Genitals

Which are the internal and which the external genitals, Doctor?

The internal sex organs include the ovaries, tubes, uterus and vagina, while the external female genitals are those which are more or less exposed. Collectively these are known as the vulva, and consist of the outer lips, the inner lips, the clitoris and the hymen. You may perhaps get a clearer understanding of the relation of these organs from this diagram (Figure 4, page 78).

The external genitals present numerous variations in contour, general appearance, size, shape and location of the component parts. The outer lips may be thick or thin, the inner lips small or elongated, the clitoris may be long or short, hooded or exposed, the hymen may be absent or may close the entrance of the vagina completely. The vulvar features of women show, therefore, a wide range of individual differences.

Mons Veneris

What part do the external genitals have in sex and reproduction?

The external genitals protect the internal structures and also serve as the main organs of erotic sensations. Above the pubic region is a cushioned area, called the mons veneris, which is covered with short, coarse hair, the pubic hair. The pubic hair is closely associated both anatomically and physiologically with the reproductive organs. It is one of the secondary sex characters both in the male and in the female, and its appearance is considered one of the first signs of the onset of puberty. In fact, the term "puberty" comes from the word "pubescent," which means hairy.

Incidentally, there is a characteristic difference in the distribution of the hair in the two sexes. In the male, the pubic hair tapers toward the umbilicus, or navel, forming a triangle with its apex pointing upward. In the female, the upper margin of the hairy surface forms a horizontal line above the mons veneris and hence is shaped like a triangle with the apex pointing downward.

Outer Labiae

The outer lips, also called the larger lips, or labiae majorae, are two elongated cushions or folds which surround and enclose the other external genital organs. They are covered by an extension of the pubic hair and serve in the main to protect the more delicate parts of the vulva which lie on the inside. In young women, especially those who have small inner lips and who have borne no children, the two outer lips may meet in the center, covering all the other structures, which cannot be seen until the outer lips are held apart. During childbearing and childbirth and with advancing age, changes occur in the contour of the outer lips so that they no longer are close together, and the other parts of the vulva may become more readily visible.

Inner Labiae

When the outer lips are drawn apart, the inner or smaller lips, called the labiae minorae, come into view. These are parallel to the outer lips and begin near the upper point of the vulva, diverging on each side like an inverted V. In size, shape, form, position and texture, the inner lips present very wide differences. They vary from two small ridges which are hardly visible to two projecting flaps of tissue which may cover up all the underlying parts and actually have to be held apart before the vaginal orifice and other structures can be seen. We have often seen labiae barely a quarter of an inch wide and we have examined women whose inner labiae measured two and a half inches in width. Between these two extremes all kinds of variations in the form and size of these structures may be found.

On their outer side the inner lips have a firm skinlike texture, but their inner surface is lined with a more delicate type of tissue. The lips are richly supplied with blood vessels, nerves and elastic tissue, so that they are sensitive to stimuli and are subject to engorgements and slight changes in size. Under proper excitation they become more tense and firm.

The Clitoris

At the upper angle of the vulva where the two inner lips meet is located the clitoris, a small but sexually important organ. Structurally the clitoris is somewhat analogous to the penis of the male except that it is diminutive in size, being only about one fourth of an inch wide. Its tip is generally rounded, resembling somewhat a small pea. It is composed largely of erectile tissue richly supplied with nerves and is very sensitive to contact and erotic stimulation.

It is interesting that the existence of the clitoris was so little known that in 1593 a man by the name of Columbus first claimed to have "discovered" it, although it was later shown that other anatomists had described the clitoris previously. It was probably also recognized from earliest times as an important seat of sexual sensations.

Can a woman tell where her clitoris is located? Can she see it or feel it?

Like the other external genital organs, the clitoris varies greatly in size and form. Sometimes it is so small and so completely covered over by extensions from the inner lips, which form a sort of hood over it, called the prepuce, that it is rather difficult to see. In many women, however, this organ is well developed and may be easily located. The size of the clitoris, incidentally, does not seem to bear any relation to the general size of the woman's body or to the strength of her sexual impulses.

What is the particular function of the clitoris, Doctor?

The clitoris is an important seat of the woman's sensuous feelings, and is very responsive to erotic stimuli. Because of its location in the vulva and its nearness to the vagina, it is subject to contact and pressure during sex play and sexual relations. In many women the sexual response can be evoked only by direct stimulation of the clitoris. During sexual excitation the clitoris may become firm and erect, but because of its small size the erection is not very distinctive or easily felt.

The Hymen

Where is the hymen located, Doctor?

At the entrance to the vagina. As you see in the diagram, the opening into the vagina lies between the lower edges of the inner labiae. In the virgin, it is partially covered by the hymen, or maidenhead. In most cases the hymen is shaped like a semicircle or crescent, projecting across the lower half of the vaginal orifice and leaving an opening above. But there are many variations in the shape of the hymen, and occasionally it surrounds the vaginal entrance almost completely, with but a small aperture at some point. Usually the opening in the hymen permits the passage of the tip of a finger, but the opening may be very small, almost pinpoint in size, or it may be large enough even before it is broken to permit the introduction of an examining instrument an inch or more in diameter.

Then the entrance to the vagina is not entirely closed by the hymen even in the virgin?

No, for even in the virgin there must be an opening for the menstrual discharge and other secretions to come through. In the rare cases where there is no opening—cases of so-called "imperforate hymen"—the membrane has to be incised at puberty, as soon as menstruation begins, in order to release the accumulated blood behind it. Such cases are very infrequent, but in the few we have seen the hymen had to be opened artificially to provide relief.

What is the specific function of the hymen, Doctor?

The biological function of the hymen is still not clearly understood. It is an interesting fact that the hymen is not found in other animals, even in the higher species, except in a very rudimentary form. It seems to be a special acquisition of the human female, and it certainly plays a much more important role as a social and moral symbol than as a useful sexual organ. Metchnikoff, in fact, regarded the hymen as one of the anatomical disharmonies in the human body. He suggested that in primitive societies when sexual relations were begun at a very early age, with the male quite immature, the hymen, by narrowing the entrance into the vagina, may have served to make sexual congress more satisfactory, but that at present, when sexual relations do not as a rule occur before maturity, the hymen has lost this purpose and function. More plausible, perhaps, is the hypothesis of Havelock Ellis that the hymen serves as an obstacle to impregnation of the young female by immature, aged or feeble males, and is therefore an anatomical expression of the admiration for force which marks the female in her choice of a mate. Even so, however, the hymen has lost any such biological function in civilized human life, where forcible impregnation of the female is a rather rare occurrence.

Is it true that the hymen is often accidentally torn as a result of athletic activities?

There is a common belief that the hymen may be injured from exercise, accidents or careless manipulation. While the membrane is often quite thin, it is rarely so thin that it could be torn during the usual athletic activities or ordinary cleansing of the genitals. It takes considerable force and pressure to cause an actual tear in the membrane. The hymen may, however, be gradually stretched or dilated by long continued manipulation of the vaginal opening. Thus, for instance, the use of the internal tampon type of protection during menstruation sometimes causes a gradual dilatation of the hymen without actual break or tear.

Is it possible to tell from the condition of the hymen whether a woman has or has not had sexual relations?

As a rule it is possible to determine from a careful examination whether a woman is a virgin or not. The opening in the hymen, however, is subject to many normal variations, and at times it is quite difficult to tell whether an enlarged or dilated orifice is a natural condition or the result of sexual contact or of some other manipulation. On the other hand, I have also seen many women in whom the hymen was still present months or even years after marriage, a condition of so-called "postmarital virginity" which we shall discuss at some other time.

Bartholin's Glands

Does the breaking of the hymen always cause pain and bleeding?

That would depend largely upon the texture, consistency and position of the hymen, and upon the size of its opening. The hymen may be thick or thin, soft or fibrous, elastic or firm. It may dilate easily under pressure, with little pain or bleeding, or it may be so resistant that it will require a surgical dilatation.

Normally, the entrance into the vagina is eased by a lubricating secretion which comes from two small glandular bodies situated one on each side of the vaginal opening. Technically these are known as Bartholin's glands, and they produce a clear, viscous fluid which becomes rather profuse under sexual stimulation. Bartholin's glands are not visible, because they lie underneath the skin, but their secretion comes to the surface through two minute openings located in the groove between the hymen and the inner labiae.

Should there normally be a discharge from the vagina?

A discharge around the external genitals may come from the vulva, the vagina, or the uterus. Under perfectly healthy conditions of the genital organs there should be no vaginal discharge, except near the time of the menstrual period. The presence of a persistent and appreciable discharge at other times may indicate some local disturbance, the nature of which can be determined only by a gynecological examination.

The Female Urethra

Last time, Doctor, you mentioned that in the male there is a close relation between the urinary and sexual organs. Is there any similar connection in the female?

If you will look at the diagram of the external genitals again (Figure 4), you will notice that between the clitoris and the entrance to the vagina there is another rather small orifice. This is the opening of the urinary canal, the urethra, through which the urine passes from the bladder. There is a marked difference in shape and function of the urethra in the two sexes. In the male, the urethra is nine inches long, is curved, passes through the length of the penis, and serves not only as a channel for the urine, but also as a passage for the seminal fluid during the ejaculation. In the female, the urethra is much shorter, only from a half inch to two inches in length, is rather straight in its course, and, except for its location, has no direct connection with the sexual or reproductive apparatus.

Then there is really no direct connection between the bladder and the vagina?

No, there is no communication between the two. Although in some instances the urethra is situated close to the vaginal entrance, even then the urinary passage is distinct from the vaginal canal. The bladder empties itself through the urethra directly to the outside, so that the urine does not come in contact with the inside of the vagina.

As a matter of fact, as you see on the diagram, there are three orifices in this area, all rather close to each other. The upper one is the opening of the urethra, or urinary canal; it is very small and sometimes can hardly be distinguished, as it lies among the folds of the external genitals. A little below it, in a straight line, is the orifice of the vagina, and about two inches below that is the opening of the anus, which leads into the rectum and the intestinal tract.

We have now considered the important internal and external female sex organs. There is one other organ, however, which might well be included in any discussion of the female reproductive system —the breasts, or mammary glands, as they are technically called.

The Breasts (Mammary Glands)

What is the relation between the breasts and the sexual system of the woman?

The breasts are the most important of the secondary sexual characteristics of the female, and their development is influenced largely by the internal secretions, or hormones, of the female sex glands. During childhood there is very little difference between the breasts of the boy and those of the girl; it is only at the onset of puberty that the breasts of the girl begin to grow and enlarge, and gradually assume the characteristic feminine form.

The primary function of the breasts is, of course, to supply the nutrient fluid, or milk, for the newborn. In addition to their secretory function, however, the breasts serve as a center for erotic sensations in the woman and play an important part in her sexual responses and reactions. The nipples, particularly, and the colored surrounding area are supplied with minute muscle fibers and elastic tissue which, under contact and sexual stimulation, contract and become erect, and serve as a zone of erotic gratification.

Ovarian Hormones

Is the development of the feminine characteristics, Doctor, caused by the hormones from the ovaries?

Yes, although there really is more than one hormone produced by the ovaries. In the woman, hormone production is very much more involved than in the man, due to the greater complexity of the female reproductive functions. The main ovarian hormone, usually referred to as estrogen or the female sex hormone, controls the development of the other genital organs and of the secondary sexual characteristics of the female, but there are also other ovarian secretions which are concerned with the processes of menstruation, pregnancy and lactation. In all these, however, there is a very marked interaction between the ovary and other glands of the body, particularly the pituitary. Recent discoveries have emphasized the importance of the pituitary gland as the activator or "motor" of the entire sexual apparatus.

Castration of the Female

What happens if the ovaries of the female are removed?

The effects of the removal of the ovaries are somewhat similar to those which follow castration in the male. The spayed female does not develop the characteristics of her sex. When this operation is performed upon immature animals, the genital organs fail to develop normally. The uterus remains infantile, the mammary glands are small, and there is a general tendency toward a more or less neuter type of appearance. In the adult animal the removal of the ovaries is often followed by a gradual atrophy of the uterus, the tubes and even of the vagina, an increased deposition of fat, the development of a lethargic disposition and a loss of sexual drive.

In the woman, the effect of removal of the ovaries would depend largely upon her age at the time of the operation: the earlier it is performed, the more marked the results. If the ovaries were removed from a girl before puberty, she would not menstruate; her genitals, including her breasts, would remain undeveloped or infantile; and she would probably not develop the normal feminine physical characteristics. When the operation is performed after puberty, the changes are less marked. Among some of the effects are sterility, cessation of the menstrual periods, a decrease in the size of the genital organs, and a tendency to a deposition of fat. The general emotional and psychic manifestations which often accompany the menopause may also ensue. It is interesting to note, however, that sexual desire may be little affected by the removal of both ovaries if this is performed after maturity. In the human female, cultural and psychological factors may be more important than hormonal activity in influencing the sex impulse, and, hence, even if both ovaries are removed after puberty the woman may continue to have normal sex desire and to participate satisfactorily in marital relations.

Transplantation of Ovaries

Have any attempts been made to transplant the ovaries from one female to another?

Yes, operations of this kind have been performed many times on animals for experimental purposes, and they have served to establish definitely the relation of the ovary to the development of the sexual characters. If a young female is deprived of her ovaries and another ovary is implanted later, the animal will go on to normal sexual growth and maturity. It is even possible to feminize certain male animals by replacing their testes with an ovary. A feminized guinea pig or rat shows the physical appearance and sexual behavior and reactions of a female. A particularly striking effect is the marked enlargement of the breasts, the feminized male guinea pig yielding milk and actually suckling young ones. Sexually he reacts like a female, and he shows definite maternal instincts toward young animals placed in his cage. A somewhat similar effect has recently been obtained by injecting certain pituitary and ovarian hormones into male animals. It would almost seem as if maternal instinct and behavior were largely the result of certain chemical stimuli.

A very interesting phenomenon of abnormal lactation is the occasional appearance of milk in the breasts of both male and female newborn children. This is ascribed to the influence of the female sex hormone, which circulates in large quantities in the blood of the mother during pregnancy and is absorbed by the growing fetus.

Have transplantations of the ovary ever been performed on women?

Yes, transplantations of ovaries from one woman to another have been performed, either for therapeutic purposes or for rejuvenation effects. On occasions when it was necessary to remove the ovaries of a woman because of some disease or abnormality, surgeons have transplanted into the abdominal muscles of such patients a part or an entire ovary from another woman to offset the effects of castration. Voronoff also engrafted ovaries from female chimpanzees into a number of aging women and reported successful rejuvenation effects. There is a great deal of skepticism, however, concerning his work and the possibility of rejuvenating senile tissues by glandular implantations.

If the ovaries are removed from a woman and another woman's ovaries implanted in her, would she be able to bear children?

No. The operation is performed only with the hope that the transplanted ovary may continue to produce hormones and thus prevent the development of symptoms of the menopause. Usually, however, these ovarian grafts gradually shrink and lose their effect. In any case, the power of reproduction could not, of course, be restored in this manner, unless the new ovary were implanted very close to the end of the Fallopian tube, but I do not know of any such experiments.

As a matter of fact, ovarian transplantations are now rarely performed, for the concentrated female hormones that have become available can be used instead.

The Female Sex Hormones

Are these female hormones obtained directly from the ovary?

When the ovarian hormones were first prepared, they were extracted from the ovarian tissues. Later, however, these hormones were obtained largely from the urine of pregnant females. The production of the ovarian hormones is greatly increased during pregnancy, and, as much of it passes out in the urine, it can be extracted from this source.

There are at least two distinct sex hormones produced by the ovaries. One is produced in the follicle in which the egg matures and is called estrogen, and the other is produced by the cells of the yellow body which fills up the follicle after ovulation has taken place, and is known as progesterone. The role of these hormones has been studied extensively, and they are now being used to correct hormonal deficiencies and to stimulate sexual and reproductive activity. Much more experimental work, however, is necessary before their value and limitations can be definitely established.

In recent years substances which possess properties similar to the female sex hormone have been produced synthetically. Their effects are very similar to those of the natural estrogens, and they have been used effectively as substitutes for the more expensive estrogens. Injections of these hormones into animals whose ovaries have previously been removed replace the functions of the ovary as far as the development of the sexual characteristics and behavior is concerned. They cause a growth of the uterus, tubes, vagina and breasts, and the appearance of normal sexual activity. In women, the ovarian hormones are frequently used during the change of life, or menopause, when the ovaries gradually cease to function. These hormones help to relieve many of the menopausal symptoms and give the woman a greater sense of well-being.

It should be stressed, however, that while there has been a great deal of publicity about the use of estrogens to delay the manifestations of the aging process, they must be used with great caution in women of menopausal age and then only under the supervision of a physician.

Shall we finish our session now and continue with our discussion next time? Let me give you the names of a few books which deal with the physiology of sex and reproduction.

Bibliography

Beach, Frank A., *Hormones and Behavior,* rev. ed. Cooper Square Publishers, 1961.

Corner, George W., M.D., *The Hormones in Human Reproduction,* rev. ed. Princeton University Press, 1947.

Guttmacher, Alan F., M.D., *Pregnancy and Birth.* Signet paperback (New American Library), 1958.

Mead, Margaret, *Male and Female.* William Morrow, 1949.

Young, William C., *Sex and Internal Secretions,* 3rd ed. William and Wilkins, 1961.

CHAPTER IV

REPRODUCTION

CHILDBEARING AND CHILDBIRTH

Let us review now how reproduction takes place—the process of conception, pregnancy and childbirth.

Asexual Reproduction

Among the primitive forms of life, such as the single-celled organisms, there is no differentiation into sexes; there are no males or females, and the methods of reproduction are correspondingly simple. For instance, when an amoeba, a common one-celled animal, reaches a certain size, it merely divides into two, and each half proceeds to grow and mature until it in turn is ready to divide. The hydra, a minute fresh-water animal, sends out small buds which soon break away from the parent and develop into mature organisms. Even a flatworm may break up into several parts, each part becoming a separate individual. These methods of reproduction do not involve any sexual mechanism, and are known as asexual modes of reproduction.

However, even in primitive life certain sexual processes have been observed. One-celled organisms, for instance, may continue to multiply asexually for many generations, but after a while they show signs of fatigue or aging, or they may have to adapt to a changing environment. Then, by a mechanism still unknown, two cells will come together, fuse for a time, and separate again. During this process of fusion, or "conjugation," as it is called, the organisms exchange some of their nuclear and cellular contents; this appears to have a rejuvenating effect upon them, permitting them to resume their asexual form of multiplication.

Sexual Reproduction

In the more highly organized forms of life, nature has evolved a method whereby only a certain specialized part of the animal takes part in the process of reproduction. Special germ cells, the sperm and the egg, are formed, and new organisms arise only from the union of these two cells. In some animals, as the earthworm or the snail, the parents are hermaphroditic—that is, both the sperm and the eggs are produced by the same individual. In most species, however, there is a differentiation into two distinct sexes, the sperm-producing male and the egg-producing female. Reproduction becomes dependent upon the union of the sex cells, and this constitutes the sexual method of reproduction.

Are there any particular advantages in this form of reproduction?

In the higher forms of life, sexual reproduction allows a longer period of development and growth for the infant before birth and better parental care later on. The most important biological advantage, however, would seem to be that the union of two different cells from two distinct parents, each cell carrying its own genes and its own potentialities, offers a greater possibility for new variations to arise and hence for the evolution of new forms of life.

In highly developed multicellular organisms such as insects, fishes, birds and mammals, differentiation is achieved by a division of different functions among the different cells that comprise the individual, and the specialization of each group of these cells to perform only one specific function. It is obviously impossible for such an individual to reproduce by splitting. Consequently, certain cells of the body differentiate and form organs which are capable of producing other specialized cells which, by meeting with similar cells of another individual of the same species, are able to create new individuals of the same type. These cells carry all the biological (genetic) information pertaining to the species.

This mechanism is the only way by which a highly complex organism can reproduce without destroying itself; it also assures the interchange of biological information between different individuals and consequently favors survival of the species through better adaptation to environmental changes and evolution.

The basis of sexual reproduction is the fusion of the sperm and the egg. The significance of this fact became known only within the last hundred years, and it is an illuminating example of the comparative recency of biological science. Sperm were first seen under the microscope by Leeuwenhoek in 1677, and the egg cells of mammals were observed in the ovaries for the first time by von Baer in 1827. Yet it was not until the end of the nineteenth century that the role which each of these elements plays in the process of reproduction was recognized. And even today the full story is still not known.

Sexual reproduction may occur either outside or inside the parental bodies. Among most aquatic animals, males and females discharge their sperm and eggs into the water, where these cells meet and unite. In several rare instances the two cells meet in a special sac, called a brood pouch, located on the outside of the body. In the sea horse, oddly enough, it is the male who possesses this brood pouch, and it is he who carries the embryos around with him until they are ready for outside life.

Insemination

In practically all higher forms of life, the meeting of the sperm and the egg occurs within the body of the female, and for this purpose physical union, or copulation, is essential. During copulation the male deposits his seminal fluid in the genital tract of the female, a process called insemination. In mammals the seminal fluid is deposited into the vaginal canal, and from there the sperm ascend the female genital tract, passing through the uterus into the tubes. This process is indicated in the diagram of Figure 5, page 94.

Vaginal Insemination

In the human, are the sperm also deposited only in the vagina?

Yes. The male ejaculates his semen into the vagina near the entrance to the uterus, and within a few seconds the sperm enter the uterine canal. When the seminal fluid is first ejaculated it is thick, but in a few minutes it liquefies. Even before this happens, some sperm have already managed to reach the opening of the uterus, and, moving rapidly, they enter the uterine body.

The Entry of the Sperm into the Uterus

Do the sperm reach the uterus so quickly because of their own motion?

The motility of the sperm is no doubt a very important factor. Sperm can travel at the rate of about one eighth of an inch in a minute, or an inch in about seven to eight minutes. However, there are probably several additional factors involved. During coitus the copulatory movements bring the cervical secretions and the ejaculated semen into close contact, and this favors the penetration of the sperm into the uterus. Once the sperm are within the uterus, the muscular movements that are normal to that organ may hasten the progression of the sperm on into the tubes.

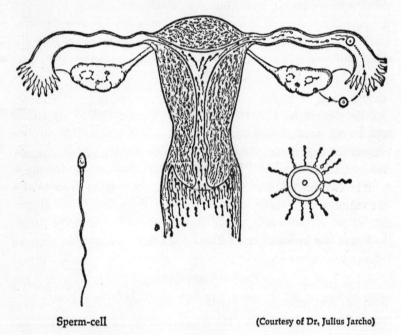

Sperm-cell   (Courtesy of Dr. Julius Jarcho)

FIGURE 5. *Sperm and Ovum in Female Genital Tract*

Do the sperm in the vagina always move toward the womb?

No, the sperm movements are aimless. Sperm move in every direction, and apparently only by chance do they reach the uterus, the tubes and the fertilization site.

Is it possible for sperm to enter the vagina while the hymen is still present? I mean, can pregnancy occur before the hymen has been broken?

Cases of pregnancy in women with intact hymens have been reported. This is very rare. It can occur only when the semen is ejaculated very close to the vaginal entrance and the woman has a copious cervical secretion which the sperm can readily penetrate.

Do all of the ejaculated sperm enter the uterus?

No, only comparatively few do. Each ejaculation contains several hundred million sperm, but only a small number of these reach and enter the uterine canal. The greater part of the ejaculate remains in the vaginal canal.

What becomes of the seminal fluid and the sperm that remain in the vagina?

Most of the fluid gradually passes out of the woman's body, although some of it may adhere to the vaginal walls for many hours. As for the sperm, they very soon become immobilized because of the hostile conditions within the vagina. Sperm cannot live in the vagina for any length of time, and the majority of them die within a few hours.

It is also possible that some of the seminal fluid is absorbed through the vaginal walls.

Would the seminal fluid absorbed in this way have any special effect upon the woman?

It has not been shown that the absorption of any part of the seminal fluid has any influence on the woman's general condition. However, some chemicals have been found in the ejaculate that when absorbed by the body of the woman will increase uterine motility. The vaginal walls have the ability to absorb many substances, including medicines; they also have the capacity to secrete fluid and with it some chemical compounds from the blood. It has been demonstrated that during sexual excitement the vaginal walls produce a serumlike fluid that may serve as lubrication during coitus.

What happens to the sperm that enter the womb? Do they remain alive in there for any length of time?

In the uterus sperm may survive for a much longer period than in the vagina, and active sperm cells have been found in the cervical canal up to seven days after intercourse. How long they can survive in the uterus and the tubes is not definitely known; however, an observer has reported them motile in the Fallopian tube as long as nine days after intercourse. It is assumed, however, that they cannot retain their fertilizing capacity for more than three days. Occasionally it has been reported thhat women became pregnant from intercourse which occurred as much as seven days before the presumed time of ovulation. Since the time of ovulation in women cannot be precisely determined, the evidence is not conclusive, and the subject requires further research.

Passage of the Sperm into the Tubes

How do the sperm reach the egg cells?

After they enter the uterus, the sperm continue moving until they come to the openings leading into the tubes. Their ascent is probably aided by the contractions of the muscles of the uterus. The sperm enter the tubes on both sides of the womb and move on. They are probably also carried along by tubal movements. If an egg is present in the tube at this time, some of the sperm will encounter it, and one of them may be able to penetrate the egg.

Fertilization

Fertilization occurs sometime after this, upon the mixing of the genetic material of both cells, which marks the moment of conception. A diagram of this is shown in Figure 6, below.

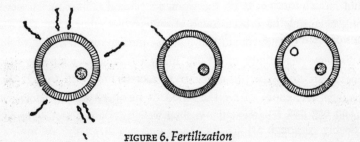

FIGURE 6. *Fertilization*

Does only one sperm enter the egg? What becomes of the others which are in the tube at the time?

Even though a large number of sperm may crowd around the egg, only one succeeds in uniting with it. As soon as this occurs, the egg membrane becomes impenetrable to other sperm. Those that remain near the egg and in other parts of the tubes disintegrate and are absorbed.

If only one sperm enters the egg, why does the ejaculate contain so many? Several hundred million, isn't it? Are such numbers necessary?

Nature seems to be quite extravagant in the number of sperm produced. However, it should be remembered that, since not all of them are able to make their way to the tubes and the fertilization site, this is probably the only way by which the survival of the species can be assured. Besides, the sperm carry with them a certain enzyme or ferment (hyaluronidase) which presumably helps to make the egg penetrable. This may be another reason why so many sperm are necessary.

How long does it take the sperm to reach the egg? I mean, how soon after intercourse can conception occur?

The length of the uterus is about three inches and that of the tubes five, making a total of about eight inches. If the sperm travel inside the body at the same rate they do when observed under the microscope, that is, an inch in seven to eight minutes, it should take them about an hour, provided they travel in a straight line and meet with no obstacles, to reach the end of the tube, where fertilization generally occurs. However, in experimental animals sperm have been recovered from the tubes twenty to thirty minutes after ejaculation, which tends to indicate that the progression of the sperm within the uterus and the tubes depends mainly on the muscular contractions of these organs.

How long does the egg last? That is, for how long is the egg capable of being fertilized?

The egg can be fertilized for only a few hours—less than a day, probably, although evidence on this point is still scanty and indirect.

What happens to the egg after it unites with the sperm?

After fertilization, the egg continues its journey toward the uterus, but its progress is rather slow, the passage through the tube taking three to four days. While in the tube, however, it already begins to develop and the initial cell begins to divide and multiply. The uterus, meanwhile, is preparing itself for the reception of the newly formed embryo. The lining of its cavity thickens and its blood supply increases to provide a suitable nesting place for the developing embryo. Within three to four days after its entry into the womb, the egg, which by now has already undergone some development, sinks deeply into this lining and, by a complicated process, gradually attaches itself. Here it continues to grow and develop until, at the end of the pregnancy, it emerges as the newborn child.

Development of the Embryo

The development of a child is certainly an amazing process.

Yes, the growth and development of the embryo, or fetus, is an extremely fascinating phenomenon, as well as a very complex one. The single cell which is formed in the tube from the fusion of the egg and the sperm soon divides into two cells which remain attached

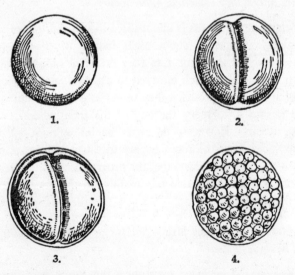

1.   2.

3.   4.

FIGURE 7. *Early Divisions of Fertilized Ovum*

to each other. Each of the two rapidly divides again, so that soon a body of four cells appears, then eight, sixteen, thirty-two and so on and on. By the time the embryo has entered the uterus from the tube, it is composed of a small ball of cells, probably the size of a pinhead. Here is a schematic drawing of the early development of the fertilized cell (Figure 7).

Later changes consist of continuous divisions of the cells and their gradual rearrangement and differentiation into various bodily structures and organs. At the end of four weeks the embryo is about one fourth of an inch in size. It is still in an unformed state, although the beginnings of facial features can now be discerned. At this time and even during the first half of the second month, the human embryo does not differ in appearance from that of other animals. In fact, it even possesses gills and exists in a sac of fluid, indicating, perhaps, the aquatic origin of life. It even has a distinct tail, which does not disappear until after the second month. By the end of the eighth week the embryo is about three quarters of an inch long, and now the human outlines become perceptible. The head, which is disproportionately large, the facial parts and the extremities can be readily distinguished. By the sixteenth week the embryo is about five inches long and possesses a definitely human form. The fingers and toes be-

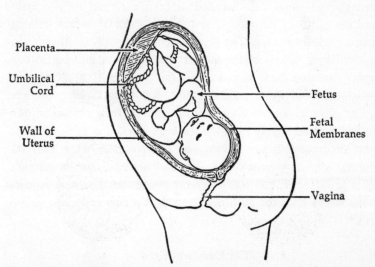

FIGURE 8. *Full-term Pregnancy. Position of fetus in uterus before birth*

come fully separated and bear soft nails, while the external genitals are already well formed so that the sex of the child can now be told. This process of growth continues until the end of the fortieth week or tenth lunal month. At the time of birth the fetus reaches a length of about twenty inches and generally weighs about seven pounds. Thus, within a period of nine months the single cell grows into a body consisting of some two hundred billion cells. A full-grown fetus within the mother's womb is shown in Figure 8, above.

The Bag of Waters

The embryo, incidentally, never lies in direct contact with the wall of the uterus during pregnancy. From the earliest stage it is surrounded by membranes which form a sac filled with the amniotic fluid, commonly referred to as the "bag of waters." In this distended sac the embryo floats rather freely at first, and the fluid serves as an excellent protective shock absorber.

The Placenta

How does the fetus get its nourishment while it is in the womb?

The cells from which the embryo obtains nourishment from its mother gradually develop into a special organ, called the placenta. Through this organ, mother and embryo maintain their contact. Here the blood of the mother and the child come in close relation without actually mixing. The placenta is like a wall which separates the circulating bloods of the mother and the fetus, but certain substances can pass both ways through this wall, and an exchange of nourishment and waste products thus takes place. During the nine months of its tenancy in the uterus the growing fetus obtains its oxygen and its food supply from the mother's blood and gives off all its waste products into her circulation. The placenta, when fully developed, is a fairly large organ. It is flattened and oval, about eight inches in diameter, and weighs over a pound. Because it is expelled by the uterus after the birth of the child, it is also called the "afterbirth."

The Umbilical Cord

The embryo is connected to the placenta by a cordlike structure, known as the umbilical cord. This cord, which is almost two feet long and about a half inch in thickness, extends from the abdomen of the fetus and contains the blood vessels which transport the fetal blood to and from the placenta. After birth the cord has to be severed in order to free the newborn child completely from its maternal attachment. The area on the baby's abdomen where the cord was originally attached remains as the navel, or umbilicus.

The uterus is normally about three inches long. How can it hold a full-grown baby?

The increase in the size of the uterus during pregnancy is due largely to an actual growth of its muscle fibers, although toward the end there is also a stretching and thinning of its walls. The uterus grows in size so that by the sixth month of pregnancy it reaches the level of the mother's umbilicus, or navel, and by the ninth it comes up nearly to the top of the abdomen. At the same time its cavity enlarges so that it can now hold from eight to ten pints of fluid. There is a corresponding increase in the weight of the organ from its usual weight of about one to two ounces to as much as two pounds at the end of pregnancy. After childbirth, however, the uterus diminishes rapidly in size and within a few weeks returns to nearly its original dimensions. This decrease is very striking, for within five or six weeks the uterus actually shrinks to one twentieth of its size at the time of childbirth.

Signs of Pregnancy

Does a woman feel anything at the time the egg is being fertilized —that is, at the moment when conception occurs?

The union of the egg and the sperm does not give rise to any feelings or sensations. Neither emotionally nor physically is the woman aware of its occurrence. It is a rather strange and often very disconcerting fact that even for the first few weeks after conception there may be neither symptoms nor signs to indicate the existence of a pregnancy. The woman may not feel any change, and a physical examination at this time may fail to disclose any evidence of conception. However, by a special urine test the presence of a pregnancy can now be determined with a fair degree of accuracy as early as four or five days after the first period has been missed.

The Urine Test for Pregnancy

Is this what they call the rabbit test? I have often wondered how the urine shows that a woman is pregnant.

No, the rabbit test for pregnancy was developed by two physicians, Aschheim and Zondek, in 1928. It depends on the presence in a pregnant woman's urine of a certain hormone produced by the placenta in rather large quantities. This hormone is capable of stimulating the ripening of the eggs in immature animals. The test itself consists in the injection of a small quantity of the woman's first morning urine into a young female mouse or rabbit. From two to three days later, depending upon the animal used, its abdomen is opened and the ovaries are examined. If the woman is pregnant, the hormones of the urine will have caused a rapid maturing of the animal's eggs, which can easily be observed by inspection of the ovaries. A certain South American male toad can also be used for the pregnancy test. When the urine of a pregnant woman is injected under the skin of this adult male toad, the hormone present will cause the toad within a few minutes to deliver a large number of sperm, which will be found in its urine.

These and other animal tests, however, have been superseded recently by the so-called immunological tests, which can be performed readily in the laboratory without involving any animals, and can produce within a few hours results of comparable accuracy.

Are these pregnancy tests reliable?

When competently performed the tests are considered to be ninety-eight per cent accurate. They are not infallible, however, and every now and then the findings prove to be incorrect. The pregnancy test cannot in itself be taken as absolute evidence of the presence or absence of a conception, but should be considered in conjunction with the other symptoms and signs of pregnancy.

How soon after conception can a woman know that she is pregnant if no urine test is taken?

The first indication of a conception is the failure of the expected menstrual period to appear. While a temporary delay of the menses may be caused by many other physical or even emotional factors, the cessation of the menses in a woman whose periods have been regular, and who has reason to believe that she may have conceived, is a presumptive sign of a pregnancy.

About two to three weeks after the expected menses have failed to appear, other symptoms of pregnancy begin to manifest themselves. There may be nausea and vomiting, called "morning sickness" because it usually occurs during the early part of the day; the breasts and nipples begin to enlarge and undergo changes in contour and coloration; there is an increased frequency of urination; the woman tends to be sleepy during the day; and she may become more sensitive emotionally. Later, after the fourth month, there is a noticeable enlargement of the abdomen, and toward the end of the fifth month the woman may begin to "feel life"—that is, she may become conscious of the movements of the fetus within her.

Is it true, Doctor, that some women continue to menstruate even after they have become pregnant?

Occasionally a pregnant woman may bleed through the vagina as though she were menstruating. However, true menstruation does not occur after pregnancy has started, and any vaginal bleeding after conception has occurred must be regarded as abnormal and be carefully investigated.

How soon after conception occurs can a doctor tell that a woman is pregnant?

The physical signs of pregnancy develop gradually, and it is not until the fifth or sixth week after conception that the enlargement of the uterus and the other genital changes suggestive of pregnancy have progressed far enough to make a diagnosis possible. Even then cases are not infrequently encountered in which it is very difficult for the physician to tell whether a woman is or is not pregnant until the eighth week or so. Later on, between the fourth and fifth months, the presence of a fetus in the uterus can be determined by means of an X ray, and during the fifth month, shortly before the woman herself begins to feel "life," the heart sounds of the baby can be heard. These are, of course, positive signs of pregnancy.

What sensations does a woman have when she "feels life"?

The feeling of "life," sometimes referred to as "quickening," is ordinarily first experienced by the woman toward the end of the fifth month of pregnancy. These sensations, when they begin, are like a gentle fluttering or tapping inside the abdomen, but gradually they become more frequent and more pronounced, although, curiously enough, they are not in the least painful or uncomfortable. The strength and frequency of the sensations depend upon the position of the baby, the thickness of the uterine wall, the amount of fluid in the sac which encloses the fetus, and other factors. The feeling of "life" can generally be taken as a definite evidence of pregnancy, although it is not an infallible symptom, for occasionally it is simulated by other internal sensations.

Can the pregnant woman feel or hear her baby's heartbeat?

No, not unless she listens to the heartbeats through a special stethoscope, an instrument used for that purpose. The sound of the baby's heart can be heard only when the ear or an instrument is placed over the mother's abdomen. The beats are rather faint, and their rate varies from 120 to 140 per minute. This is nearly twice as fast as the mother's own heartbeat, which normally ranges between seventy and eighty to the minute. It is a strange fact that it was only in the last century—in 1818, to be exact—that the fetal heart sounds were described for the first time.

False Pregnancies

As I mentioned, the presence of the fetal heartbeat can be regarded as absolute evidence of pregnancy, for this is one of the few signs which cannot be duplicated by other conditions. The extent to which a woman may occasionally show most of the other signs of pregnancy without actually being pregnant is, at times, truly remarkable. The menses may cease, nausea and vomiting may occur, the breasts may increase in size, the abdomen may enlarge to considerable proportions, and the woman may even "feel life"—and yet she may not be pregnant. All these symptoms may be simulated by emotional factors and by conditions unrelated to pregnancy. The uterus, of course, does not enlarge, and the feeling of "life" is caused by the movement of gas in the intestines. Such cases of "false pregnancy" occur mainly in elderly women who are very anxious to have a child, but instances have been reported in younger women too. Such imaginary pregnancies are comparatively rare.

To what extent does the health of the mother influence the child within her?

It is perhaps well to emphasize that the embryo in the uterus is in reality not a part of the mother. At the moment of the fusion of the sperm and the egg a new life comes into being. The mother provides the embryo with protection and nourishment, but its development goes on quite independently. In other words, within the fertilized egg are already packed all the innumerable physical and mental qualities and characteristics of the child-to-be, and these are but little influenced by the experiences of the mother during the period of pregnancy.

Prenatal Influences

The physical growth and development of the fetus, however, do depend to a considerable extent upon the supply of food materials which comes to it through the mother's blood, and the diet of the mother may thus indirectly influence the condition of the baby. During wars, for instance, infants born in countries where the food supply is meager are often significantly below the average in weight and size at birth. The physical condition of the mother during her pregnancy may thus have a definite influence upon the well-being of the coming offspring. In general, however, if there is not sufficient nourishment for both the mother and the developing child the child receives the available nourishment and the deficiency is borne by the mother.

Does the emotional state of a pregnant woman affect the unborn child in any way?

Passing moods and temporary emotional strains in a pregnant woman have no known influence upon the child within her. Severe or lasting emotional disturbances, however, may indirectly affect the mother's glandular balance and her general physical condition, and thus also affect the growing baby.

Birthmarks

Can a scare or a shock during pregnancy leave a physical impression upon the child?

Although many women connect the presence of certain skin marks on a child with some disturbing incident during the course of the pregnancy, there is no basis for the assumption that any sudden experience on the part of the mother will leave a physical mark upon the child.

How long does pregnancy last? How much time elapses from the day of conception until the birth of the child?

The average duration of pregnancy, from the time of conception until birth, is about 266 days. In figuring the expected day of childbirth, however, the calculations are made from the first day of the last menstruation, since this date is known, while the exact time of conception can only be approximated. Accordingly, childbirth should be expected 280 days—which is ten lunar months, or about nine calendar months—from the first day of the last menstrual flow. There are, however, wide individual variations, and only about one pregnancy in ten ends exactly 280 days from the start of the last menstruation. Hence it is seldom possible to predict accurately the date of an expected childbirth.

Childbirth

What makes labor start?

The factors which cause the child to be born have long been a puzzling medical problem. Even today it is not clearly understood whether the onset of labor is due to changes in the life processes of the fetus itself or in those of the mother. Many theories have been offered to account for this phenomenon, but none of them have proven entirely adequate. However, in all species, whether the fetus weighs a few grams or several hundred pounds, as in the elephant, labor regularly begins at a specific time—namely, when the fetus is sufficiently mature to cope with extra-uterine conditions, but not large enough to cause mechanical difficulties in delivery. The factors regulating this highly synchronized sequence of events are obscure.

The initiation of childbirth has been attributed to the action of certain hormones secreted by the pituitary gland which have the effect of increasing uterine contractility; also to the mechanical effect of the distension of the uterus by the fetus and the amniotic fluid reaching a point at which the organ is unable to distend any farther and therefore tries to rid itself of its contents. However, the theory presently in vogue is that labor starts by a diminution of one of the hormones produced by the placenta. This hormone has a blocking effect upon the uterine muscle fibers, preventing them from contracting in a synchronous way. As the production of this hormone diminishes, the blocking effect disappears and labor starts. This theory, although the most popular, is still contested.

How long does the process of childbirth take?

The duration of labor depends upon the size of the child, the pelvic dimensions of the mother, the contractile powers of her uterine muscles, her general condition and a number of other factors. The average period of labor is about sixteen hours for a firstborn, and about ten hours for subsequent births. The process is generally divided into several stages. The first stage extends from the beginning of the uterine contractions, which mark the onset of labor, until the time when the opening of the cervix is dilated sufficiently to permit the passage of the child. The dilation occurs in part as a result of the mechanics of the muscular action of the uterus itself, and in part through the pressure of the "bag of waters" which surrounds the baby. As the uterus contracts above, this bag is forced downward and acts like a wedge which aids materially in dilating the opening. When the dilatation is nearly complete, the bag breaks and the fluid runs out. The usual duration of the first stage varies from nine to fourteen hours.

During the second stage, the child is expelled from the uterus and is forced through the vagina to the outside. Usually the head comes out first and then the rest of the body soon follows. The pains are stronger and more frequent during this period, but this stage lasts only about two hours or less. Even after the child emerges, it is still attached to the mother by the umbilical cord, which extends from its abdomen to the placenta in the uterus. This cord has to be severed to free the child completely from its maternal attachment.

The third stage of labor consists of the expulsion of the placenta and the membranes which had surrounded the fetus. This occurs usually about half an hour or so after the birth of the child, hence the name "afterbirth." The pains during this stage are comparatively mild and of short duration.

What is "dry labor"? I have heard it spoken of in connection with childbirth.

As I mentioned, the sac of fluid, or bag of waters, in which the baby lies, usually breaks toward the end of the first stage of labor —that is, when the opening of the uterus is almost fully dilated. It may happen, however, that the bag breaks much earlier, at the very beginning of labor or even before its onset. As the fluid runs out at this time, the subsequent childbirth is sometimes referred to as a "dry labor." Because the dilating effect of the water bag is thereby lost, the delivery may become a little more difficult and prolonged.

Does the baby always come out of the mother head first?

No, not always, but in the majority of instances. In about ninety-six per cent of all cases, the head is the first part to appear during birth. The usual position of the fetus in the womb is with its head downward and with its arms and legs bent or flexed, in order to occupy the least space. As the head points down, it will naturally be the first part to emerge during labor, and the child is therefore generally born in this position. Because of its rounded shape and its comparative firmness, the head also serves as an excellent aid in dilating the uterine opening during childbirth. The child may, however, lie in a different position, and the part to appear first may be the face, the extremities, or the buttocks. In about three per cent of deliveries, the buttocks are the first to appear, followed by the legs. Such cases are referred to as "breech" deliveries and carry a slightly greater risk to the infant. It is quite common, however, for the baby to be in breech position during the greater part of pregnancy and then change its position to a head presentation as the day of confinement nears.

The first instinctive act of the newborn baby is to cry. The transition from the protected and warm surroundings of the mother's womb to the colder outside environment constitutes a profound change in the life of the infant. Upon birth its communication with the circulation of the mother is interrupted, and it is no longer able to obtain its food and oxygen from that source. With the cry the newborn infant expands its lungs and establishes its own respiration so that it may take in the oxygen directly from the outside air.

Painless Childbirth

But why is childbirth so painful, Doctor? It would seem that such a normal function shouldn't be accompanied by so much distress.

Well, childbirth need not necessarily be a painful process. Among primitive peoples, and even among agricultural peoples today who marry young, childbirth is reported to be comparatively simple. Here, for instance, is the story of a childbirth episode in the home of a Balkan peasant as reported by an observer a few years ago. The woman was making bread; she had set some loaves to bake, and went to the shed for more wood. While she was collecting the wood she suddenly felt a stab of pain. The baby was already on its way, and it was born immediately. She tied the cord herself and cut it with her pocketknife. She then called her mother-in-law, who came in and carried the baby into the house, while she herself remained in the shed until the afterbirth came away. That day she did no more work, but the next day she was about as usual. In India I found that anesthetics are rarely used in childbirth and that most women in the villages deliver their babies with little complaint. This is true of peasant women in other countries as well.

Many factors are responsible for this ease of childbearing and childbirth among primitive peoples and among agricultural populations generally. The woman has ample sunshine on her exposed body and her diet contains the essential vitamins, so that her skeleton and pelvis are well developed. At the same time, her hard and active life tends to diminish the size of her child, so that labor is so much easier for her. There is also little mixture of racial types, and the bones and organs of the mother are well suited for the type of child she is to bear. The woman whose pelvis, for instance, is adapted for a long-headed baby is usually impregnated by a man of her own type, and not by one of a different race who might transmit to the offspring a wide head or larger body. Then, again, she is mentally and emotionally much more placid and accepts her role in childbearing more naturally.

In our urban and industrialized culture childbirth is not so simple. It is true that physically women are constituted to have children, but this function is not necessarily perfect. Pregnancy and childbirth involve certain muscles which in present-day life are not as well developed as they should be for efficient functioning. Furthermore, the emotional tensions to which we are constantly subjected also have an adverse influence upon the normal function of our muscles. Fear in itself is able to cause marked bodily changes, and in our culture, at least, women are conditioned to look forward to childbirth with a great deal of apprehension and anxiety. As a result of these factors, the process of bringing forth children has become considerably more difficult in our civilization.

What can be done to ease labor pains?

During the first hours of labor the pains are comparatively mild; it is only in the later stages that the pains may become quite severe. With present-day obstetrical care, however, even these can be largely relieved by the administration of sedatives or anesthetics, or by the resort to various physical and psychotherapeutic measures.

What about "natural childbirth"? Is it really painless?

Many obstetricians encourage their patients to deliver by what is called natural childbirth. Natural childbirth is not altogether without pain, but it is without fear. It might perhaps better be called fearless childbirth.

There is no human experience comparable to the satisfaction of a woman giving birth in full consciousness to a wanted child. A loving couple cherish the thought of the coming child throughout pregnancy; the long months are full of love, joy and expectation. If the obstetrician is able to gain the confidence of both husband and wife, he may be able to dispel their fears of a painful delivery and the uncertainties that attend it. With warm understanding and reassurance, he must engage their cooperation. The woman is prepared through discussion to face childbirth without the usual tensions and anxieties and, through the special breathing and physical exercises, to relax and prepare her body for the event. This makes it possible for her to cope more readily with the discomforts of birth. She will learn what to expect and what will be expected of her. She should know that her obstetrician will be present, that he will help her throughout the delivery, and that if the need arises she will receive adequate sedation or medication.

If she is physically and emotionally well-prepared, she may be able to go through childbirth fully conscious and give birth by her own effort. Such an event will give her a profound sense of satisfaction and exaltation.

Is it not true that sometimes instruments are necessary to deliver a child?

Sometimes, as when the contractions of the uterine muscle are not strong enough, the obstetrician may have to help the baby out of the womb. He will use a special instrument, known as forceps, which consists of two metal parts curved so as to fit the baby's head. As a rule forceps are employed only in the second stage of labor, when the baby's head is about to emerge from the vagina, and they provide a useful mechanical means for helping a mother when labor is prolonged and difficult. Forceps are not used, however, without some form of anesthesia.

Caesarean Operation

When is it necessary to operate on the mother and remove the child through the abdomen?

The procedure you refer to is called a Caesarean operation or section. First the abdomen is opened, then the uterus, and the child is extracted through the incision. This operation has been practiced from earliest time, but until the fourteenth or the fifteenth century it was performed only on women who had died in labor, in an attempt at least to save the child. In 715 B.C. a law was enacted in

Rome which prescribed that the child should be removed in this manner from any woman who died during the last few weeks of her pregnancy; as the Roman laws later became known as the laws of Caesar, it is assumed that the name "Caesarean operation" originated at the time. There is also a legend, though, that Julius Caesar was delivered through an abdominal incision, and that the operation was therefore named after him.

The modern type of operation was first described in 1882, by the German physician Sanger, and since then it has been improved and perfected to a remarkable degree. It is usually performed wherever a safe delivery in a less radical manner is not possible. With the modern improvements in techniques, the operation has lost practically all of its dangers, and it is resorted to with increasing frequency in difficult labors for the purpose of saving the life and health of both mother and child.

Extra-uterine Pregnancies

I have heard that a pregnancy can occur outside the womb. Is this true?

Ordinarily, as we saw, the union of the egg and the sperm occurs in the outer part of the tube, and then the fertilized egg makes its way slowly down the tube until it finally reaches the uterus and lodges there. It may happen, however, that this journey to the uterus is interfered with and the egg is stopped at some point of its route. Inflammations of the tube, constrictions along its walls, or anatomical abnormalities of its structure are among the more common causes of such a condition. At any rate, instead of entering the uterus, the fertilized egg attaches itself to the tubal wall and commences to grow and develop there. This is called an extra-uterine or ectopic pregnancy, and usually requires operative interference.

Can a woman herself tell when a pregnancy occurs outside the womb?

No. The symptoms of an extra-uterine pregnancy are at first indefinite, and it may be difficult even for a physician to establish a diagnosis during the first few weeks. Frequently the history is that a woman who has missed a menstrual period, and who shows the usual early manifestations of pregnancy, begins to notice some irregular vaginal bleeding or staining and perhaps also experiences cramplike pains in the lower abdomen on one or the other side. A gynecological examination at this time may reveal indications of the abnormal location of the pregnancy.

What would happen if the pregnancy were to go on? Would it be dangerous for the woman?

There is the danger that the wall of the tube may break at any moment and cause a serious internal hemorrhage. When a definite diagnosis of a tubal pregnancy is made, it is always necessary to operate and remove the developing egg before complications arise. It is extremely unlikely for a living child to result from an extra-uterine pregnancy, although a few cases have been reported where, after rupture of the tube, the embryo attached itself to some part of the abdomen and continued to develop to full term.

Hasn't modern civilization made childbearing more dangerous than it used to be?

Not at all. It is well to bear in mind that formerly whenever any abnormal complication arose during childbirth, both the mother and the child almost inevitably perished, and numberless women died because of infections and unsanitary care. While the modern civilized woman has greater difficulty in childbirth, the progress of obstetrical science and technique has served to save a very great number of women and children who would not have survived under more primitive conditions. Both maternal and infant mortality have been greatly reduced in most countries during the past half century.

The Lying-in Period

After a woman has given birth, how long does it take before her organs return to their normal condition?

Pregnancy influences profoundly not only the reproductive organs but the entire system of the woman, and the actual process of labor affects the tissues of the genital tract. The cervix, the vagina and the vulva are stretched and distended to a very marked degree during the passage of the baby. All these changes, however, are only temporary, and the period of repair and involution is remarkably rapid. Within six to eight weeks after a normal delivery the generative organs of the woman return to nearly their original condition. Difficult labors, however, may result in a more permanent stretching and relaxation of the muscles of the genital tract, a condition which may require surgical repair.

How long should a woman remain in bed after her confinement?

The lying-in period—that is, the length of time a woman should rest after her delivery—varies according to the type of delivery, her general physical condition and the rapidity with which her organs recover. Peasant women may be back at work in two or three days or even within a few hours after labor. Whereas two weeks used to be the length of the recommended hospital stay, patients nowadays are allowed out of bed sometimes within hours after delivery, and in some places the woman even walks to her bed from the delivery room. The hospital stay for a normal delivery usually lasts from three days to a week, during which the woman is encouraged to leave her bed and walk as soon as she can.

This accelerated program helps recovery to normal, although it does not mean that a woman is able to resume all her usual activities immediately upon returning home. Her organs and her body need to recover from the nervous and physical strains of the months of pregnancy and to adjust to the feeding and care of the new baby in the home. She should avoid strenuous exertion and plan for naps or bed rest at frequent intervals. If possible, extra help should be secured for the first few weeks at home.

How soon after the child is born does milk appear in the mother's breasts?

During pregnancy the woman's breasts enlarge in preparation for their new function. The first secretion of the breasts is colostrum, a fluid much thicker than and different from milk; it appears about the first or second day after delivery. Milk secretion begins in the second to fourth day. Breast feeding, which had been out of fashion, is being encouraged again, since it is certain that there is no better food for the child. Generally, any woman who sincerely wishes to breast-feed her child is able to do so. In some cases it may require a little extra effort and patience and the cooperation of her physician. Breast feeding has been proved to provide greater emotional security for the child and a better relationship between the child and the mother. It has also been shown that women who nurse their children are less susceptible to later cancer of the breast.

Breast feeding should continue for about six months, although many women prefer to continue longer, and some, due to other obligations, must shorten this time. Prolonging lactation beyond a year has not proved to be physically desirable, either for the mother or for the child.

How soon after childbirth can sexual relations be resumed?

When the woman leaves the hospital, her organs are far from normal. Her uterus and its opening are still somewhat enlarged, and a bloody vaginal discharge will continue for some days. There is a serious possibility of infection if sexual relations are resumed at this time. Consequently, it is advisable to wait until the discharge has stopped and the obstetrician's check-up examination has been performed.

In any event, total abstinence is usually recommended for six to eight weeks after childbirth.

Is contraception necessary during the nursing period?

Many women believe that pregnancy cannot occur while they are nursing, for the reestablishment of normal menstruation is delayed during this period. However, pregnancy can occur before the reappearance of menses if no contraception is used. Women who wish to space their children should start using contraception at the time of resuming sexual relations.

How soon after delivery does a woman begin to menstruate again?

That depends largely on whether the mother is nursing her baby or not. If she is, menses may appear as early as the second month or as late as the eighteenth following delivery; usually it is between three and four months. If she is not nursing, menses usually reappear within three months.

Twins

What about twins?

Twins or other multiple births may come about in two different ways. Ordinarily only one egg ripens and comes out of the ovary during the month. It is possible, however, for two or more eggs to ripen in the same month, either in one or both of the ovaries. All these eggs may be fertilized at the same time, and the woman will then give birth to twins, triplets, quadruplets or even quintuplets, as the case may be. Each embryo develops quite independently within its own sac and with its own attachments to the uterus. Such children come from separate eggs and separate sperm, and they resemble each other no more than do other brothers and sisters. They may be of different sexes and may be quite unlike each other physically, mentally and temperamentally.

Twins, however, may also come from but a single fertilized egg. Soon after fertilization, the egg ordinarily divides into two cells which remain attached to each other. In some instances, though, these two cells, instead of remaining attached, fall apart, and each one continues to develop independently of the other. When both of them go on to complete maturity, twins are born, but such twins coming originally from a single fertilized egg are very much alike in every respect. They are of the same sex, they possess similar physical and mental traits, and are known as identical twins.

Is it true that the bearing of twins is apt to run in families?

Twinning often occurs in several members of the same family, and there is considerable evidence that the tendency is hereditary. Some women, furthermore, tend to have multiple births at each pregnancy. There is the authenticated record, for instance, of a woman who had three unrelated husbands, and with each one of them she had twins, triplets, and with one even quadruplets; in fifteen pregnancies she gave birth to forty-two children. This woman's fertility obviously could not be ascribed to any particular quality on the part of her husbands. On the other hand, there is the story of the Russian peasant whose two successive wives gave birth to twins and triplets, so that he had a total of eighty-seven children to his credit. This might indicate that the male too may carry the quality of multiple births within him. Aside from the hereditary factor, however, twinning is more apt to occur in women between the ages of thirty-five and forty than in younger women, and it is also more prevalent in northern than in southern countries.

Is it possible to tell during pregnancy whether a woman is carrying twins?

In the early months it may be difficult to determine the presence of twins. In the latter months, however, the more marked abdominal enlargement and the detection of the outlines of two different bodies may serve to indicate the presence of more than one embryo. A definite diagnosis of twins can be made when two distinct fetal hearts are heard on examination. The rate at which the two hearts beat is very rarely the same, and when the doctor hears, for instance, at one point a fetal heart beating at a rate of 120 times per minute and at another point a heart beating 140 times a minute, it is certain that there are two different embryos in the uterus. The presence of twins can also be diagnosed by means of X rays, which would show the outlines of two distinct fetal bodies.

How often do twins occur?

Twinning varies widely among different races and perhaps also in different climates. It is most frequent among Negroes and least frequent among yellow races. In the United States, the frequency of twinning for the white population is one in ninety-three births, whereas for the Negro population it is one in seventy-three. In Japan, the frequency of twinning is about half that of the United States—one in 155 births.

I have heard that new drugs that are used to promote fertility have resulted in multiple births.

One of the problems encountered in couples unable to conceive is that some women do not ovulate. Several new preparations are being studied to overcome this problem. There is a chemical which you may have heard of (Clomid), and also extracts of the pituitary gland as well as of the urine of menopausal women; some of these drugs are still in the experimental stage, and some may not ever become available to all physicians. The use of these drugs has been associated occasionally with multiple births. The reason for this is that it is impossible for even the most experienced medical investigator to know the exact sensitivity of a woman's ovaries to such stimulation at any particular time.

What is the largest number of children ever born to a woman at one time?

Seven is the largest reported number born at one time. However, there is not a single report of children surviving a multiple delivery of more than five for any appreciable length of time. Multiple pregnancies and deliveries seem to be occurring oftener, but this may be due only to better reporting and communications.

Incidentally, the mortality rate of quadruplets and triplets is very high, as practically all of them are born prematurely and may die soon after birth. A high percentage of twin pregnancies also end before term.

Sex Prediction

Can the sex of a child be told before its birth?

Yes; nowadays it is possible to tell the sex of the baby before birth by studying the cells found in the amniotic fluid. Of course, this cannot be done routinely, since a definite risk to the pregnancy is involved in obtaining a sample of this fluid. However, occasionally the course of the pregnancy may oblige the obstetrician to perform some intra-uterine studies, during the course of which a sample of the amniotic fluid can be obtained. When stained by a special dye, some of the cells in the fluid will show a small body attached to the nuclear membrane. This body is found in much higher proportion in females than in males and is called the "nuclear sex." A study of it makes it possible to state the sex even when the embryo is too small to show any sex differentiation.

Sex Determination

What determines the sex of the offspring?

The sex of the offspring is determined by the particular type of sperm that happens to fertilize the ovum; the sperm are of two types, one male-producing and the other female-producing, which apparently are formed in equal numbers.

Then the mother really plays no part in the determination of the sex of the child?

Not as far as our present knowledge indicates.

Is there anything that can influence the sex of the child after a pregnancy has already started?

No. Sex is established at the moment of conception and, as we have already said, by the type of sperm that fertilizes the egg. There is no possibility at all of changing the sex of the offspring at any stage. Some hormones if given to the mother during pregnancy may alter the appearance of the sex organs of the child to a degree that may make sex assignment difficult. In such a case, a study of the nuclear sex should immediately be made in order to dispel any doubt.

Is there any way, then, by which the sex of the child may be controlled?

Not at present. Many stories have been published suggesting this possibility, and quack treatments have been tried to achieve the conception of a baby of a desired sex. None of the reported attempts has any scientific basis. Theoretically, it is possible that when a way is found to separate male-producing from female-producing sperm the sex of the child might be predetermined by selective artificial insemination of sperm of the desired sex.

Bibliography

Dick-Read, Grantly, M.D., *Natural Childbirth Primer*. Harper paperback, 1956.
Eastman, Nicholson J., M.D., *Expectant Motherhood*, 4th rev. ed. Little, Brown, 1963.

Flanagan, Geraldine, *The First Nine Months of Life.* Simon and Schuster, 1962.

Gilbert, Margaret S., *Biography of the Unborn,* 2nd rev. ed. Hafner, 1963.

Guttmacher, Alan F., *Pregnancy and Birth.* Signet paperback (New American Library), 1958.

Hartman, Carl G., *Science and the Safe Period: A Compendium of Human Reproduction.* Williams and Wilkins, 1962.

Kaufman, Sherwin A., M.D., *The Ageless Woman.* Prentice-Hall, 1967.

Power, Jules, *How Life Begins.* Simon and Schuster, 1965.

Robinson, J. F., *Having a Baby,* 3rd ed. Williams and Wilkins, 1966.

CHAPTER V

FAMILY PLANNING

Before we continue today, is there any phase of reproduction which you would like me to clarify further?

Yes, there is one closely related subject which we'd very much like to discuss with you—the question of birth control. As we said to you once, Doctor, we both want children. Just now, however, we are not in a position to plan for a baby, at least not for the next year or two, and we should not want to have one until we can afford to give the child proper care and a decent upbringing. In the meantime, we shall, of course, have to consider the question of birth control, and we'd like to talk to you about it now.

Birth Control and Health

Very well. I shall be glad to discuss with you the problems of family planning and the control of conception, for they are a very significant aspect of the marital relation. Birth control is still, as you know, a controversial topic, which carries with it many social, economic, political, religious, and moral implications that provoke a wide and sincere divergence of opinion. However, a substantial change has occurred in the last few years, and a more tolerant attitude toward birth control is rapidly becoming widespread. In my opinion, parenthood should not be left to chance. It is an important decision for any couple. Let us, however, consider the question primarily from a medical point of view.

The planning of parenthood constitutes, in my opinion, an important individual and social health measure, for it helps to conserve the well-being of the parents, the family and the home. I am not speaking merely of women who should not bear children because of some illness; obviously, if a woman is suffering from an ailment—whether of body or mind—which would make a pregnancy hazardous for her, she must be given adequate contraceptive information as a therapeutic measure. But even when she is in good health, she should learn how to space her children in order to preserve her future well-being. Not many women, in our culture and under our present mode of life, can or want to go on bearing children to the limit of their reproductive capacity. Nor is it good for the child to be born too close to its sister or brother. From a medical viewpoint, too frequent pregnancies without sufficient intervals are to be avoided for the sake of both the mother and the child. Then again, the recurrent fear of an unwanted pregnancy makes a satisfactory marital adjustment difficult to attain. Hence some knowledge of the means of controlling conception should be a part of preparation for marriage.

Medical Indications for Birth Control

What conditions would make it inadvisable for a woman to bear children?

Nowadays, medicine has progressed to such a degree that almost any woman, regardless of her physical condition, can carry a pregnancy to term. However, there are some medical conditions which make a pregnancy hazardous to the woman. Certain diseases of the heart, for instance, or of the kidneys, tuberculosis, diabetes, previous Caesarean sections, or even certain types of psychopathic disorders may make childbearing or childbirth dangerous. Under such circumstances the use of birth-control measures becomes medically necessary to conserve the health or even to preserve the life of the woman.

Eugenic Indications

The use of contraception may also become necessary for eugenic reasons. When either the husband or the wife suffers from a physical or mental disorder that might be transmitted to offspring, childbearing may have to be avoided.

Spacing of Children

Then there is the question of the spacing of children. It is quite generally accepted that there should be a definite interval between successive childbearings. Lack of proper spacing of births has a deleterious effect both upon the mother and upon her offspring, as has been shown by a number of statistical studies. The New York Academy of Medicine, one of the leading medical bodies in this country, recommends that "child spacing should be recognized as a medical indication" for giving contraceptive advice.

Would you say, then, that every married couple should be given information about family planning?

I think that every couple should receive adequate information about the prevention of conception, preferably as preparation for marriage. They should be provided with whatever knowledge is available to make it possible for them to plan their future family in an intelligent manner. Most American couples today resort to contraceptive practices of one kind or another with the aim of regulating childbearing. All too often they do not have adequate information about the different methods available or about how to avoid practices which are either unreliable, harmful or unsatisfactory.

Birth Control and Morality

Some people argue that any attempt to prevent conception is unnatural, and that those who use birth control "conspire to cheat the laws of nature."

Most of the achievements of civilization have been made possible by man's learning how to control the forces of nature. The use of the lightning rod, of steam heat, of anesthesia during childbirth, are all unnatural in the sense that they tend to interfere with natural phenomena or to "cheat the laws of nature," yet we should hardly wish to do without them. The practice of birth control is but another step in the increase of our power to control human welfare rationally. Few people nowadays deny the need for family planning; it is only a question as to what particular method should be employed for the purpose of controlling conception.

But isn't it against certain religious tenets to use measures to avoid conception?

Some people sincerely believe that the sexual union should serve primarily the purpose of procreation, and that it is sinful to avoid or prevent conception while continuing marital relations. Yet this is not the position even of church authorities today. In the main, present religious opinion looks upon family planning as a social responsibility entirely in harmony with ethical and moral beliefs. In a report on this subject by the Federal Council of Churches, for instance, the following statement appears:

A majority of the committee hold that the careful and restrained use of contraceptives by married people is valid and moral. They take this position because they believe that it is important to provide for the proper spacing of children, the control of the size of the family and the protection of mothers and children; and because intercourse between mates, when an expression of their spiritual union and affection, is right in itself.

Primitive Birth Control

Did primitive peoples also try to regulate the size of their families or is it a modern idea?

The idea of family regulation is not new. From time immemorial man has been endeavoring consciously to control the number of his offspring. In fact, among certain primitive societies failure to exercise moderation in the size of one's family was even regarded as a manifestation of unpardonable improvidence. The means employed by these peoples to limit the number of their children were generally very much more drastic than our own. Unwanted babies were often left exposed or were destroyed, infanticide being a widespread practice. Later, when man learned that, instead of destroying the child after birth, it was possible to destroy the products of conception before birth, abortion came into wide use, and it is still all too often resorted to today.

With the growth of human knowledge, however, and with an increase in the understanding of the physiology of reproduction, man found that in order to regulate the size of the family it was not necessary to destroy the child either before or after its birth, but that it was possible to control parenthood by preventing conception. Thus we come to what is obviously the most intelligent, most rational and most humane method for family regulation.

The Modern Planned-Parenthood Movement
Did they also use birth-control measures in primitive times?

Yes, even among primitive groups various methods of contraception were employed, although these were generally very crude and naïve. The primitive woman relied mainly upon weird potions and concoctions, or upon magical incantations and charms, which were supposed to render her sterile. Or else taboos on sexual relations under various circumstances served as a means of preventing conception. References to the use of birth-control measures can be found in the medical and lay literature of every period. A prescription for a contraceptive preparation was even discovered in an Egyptian papyrus which dates back some four thousand years. Malthus published his *Essay on Population,* a book which served as the impetus for the family-limitation movement, in 1798, and a complete medical volume on contraception, *The Fruits of Philosophy,* was published by an American physician, Dr. Knowlton, in 1832—well over a hundred years ago. It is quite true, however, that the widespread interest in family planning is comparatively recent in origin. It was only in the early part of this century that Margaret Sanger first began to advocate a wider dissemination of birth-control knowledge and initiated the birth-control movement in this country. And only now is the significance of family regulation as a crucial factor in human welfare and in national and international relations becoming widely recognized. The rapid social, economic and political changes of our age are making family planning an essential need in modern life.

Voluntary Parenthood
Some people think that if birth-control knowledge were freely available many would avoid the responsibility of marriage and children altogether.

To have children is a normal desire in mature people, and this desire impels responsible individuals to start a family within the framework of marriage. Information about contraception does not in the least diminish this desire. It merely enables parents to regulate the time of childbearing and the number of their offspring in accordance with their particular circumstances. The use of contraceptive measures makes a pregnancy a matter of deliberate planning rather than the mere accidental result of a sexual relation. Children should certainly come by choice rather than by chance. Planned and wanted children have a better chance from the start for adequate physical and emotional development.

Sexual relations cannot be restricted to those few occasions when conception is desired. Free sex expression between spouses consolidates and strengthens the marriage bond.

Among animals, sexual contact occurs only at the time when the female is susceptible to fertilization. Only at this time will the female readily accept the male, and only at this time will the male be aroused by the female. In human life, the sexual relation serves an additional purpose in marriage—it adds an essential physical and spiritual unity and balance to the association of the man and the woman. This balance is damaged or destroyed when the constant fear of unwanted pregnancy is present.

How long is it desirable to wait between one pregnancy and the next?

That would depend to a large degree upon the health of the individual woman, the number and character of her previous pregnancies and labors, and many other factors. Even in the case of a perfectly healthy woman, however, an interval between successive childbearings is desirable. Each couple should decide which is the best interval for them. However, in general, medical opinion advises spacing children at least two years apart.

Continence

What about self-control? Would it be advisable for people to abstain altogether from sexual relations when a pregnancy is not desired?

Continence is occasionally resorted to for the purpose of preventing conception, and there are records of couples who have abstained from sexual contact even for years at a time. There is no health problem in avoiding sexual relations for a long period of time, but most people would find it very difficult to adjust to this discipline.

When two people who love each other and live together in the close intimacies of marriage attempt to avoid sexual relations, it inevitably gives rise to marked physical stresses and emotional strains, which are very likely to lead to serious disharmonies and marital conflicts. A satisfactory sex life is essential for a satisfactory marital union, and not many marriages can long survive the complete repression of the sexual instinct.

The "Safe Period"

What about the rhythm method? Aren't there certain days during a woman's menstrual month when she is safe and cannot become pregnant?

Yes, there is a rhythm of fertile and infertile days in the woman's menstrual month. Impregnation can occur only on certain days of the cycle. During the other days sexual relations are not apt to result in conception. This constitutes the "rhythm," or "safe-period," method of conception control.

The belief that there is a period in the menstrual cycle during which conception is not possible probably dates back to antiquity. Over two thousand years ago Hindu physicians spoke of a period of absolute sterility in the menstrual month. The Mosaic laws which prohibit sexual relations during the menstrual flow and for a week thereafter were possibly based on the theory that certain days of the month were more likely to be fertile. Soranus, a Greek physician who practiced in Rome during the second century, advised women who wanted to prevent conception to limit their sexual relations to certain periods of the month. In more recent times, Capellmann, in a book published in 1883, mentioned specific days as being free from the chance of conception and advocated this safe period as a means of birth control. The days he mentioned, however, have since been shown to be quite incorrect. Advances in knowledge of the physiology of reproduction, particularly the investigations of Knaus of Austria and Ogino of Japan, have given a new impetus to the study of the subject. These two physicians charted the fertile and sterile days of the menstrual month and established the existence of a "safe period" on a more scientific basis. This method of family limitation has received the sanction and endorsement of Catholic authorities.

The Physiological Basis of the "Safe Period"

What is the scientific explanation of the safe period?

It is generally accepted that in the human female only one egg is released each month, and that the egg retains its vitality—that is, its capacity to be fertilized—only for a short time, a few hours at the most. Hence, unless the egg is fertilized soon after its release from the ovary, impregnation becomes impossible until the next ovulation a month later.

The sperm, although they are able to survive for several days, lose their fertilizing power long before they die. It is generally accepted that they may be able to fertilize an egg up to seventy-two hours after entering the uterus. As I said earlier, there have been occasional reports of women becoming pregnant from intercourse which occurred as much as seven days before the presumed time of ovulation, but the evidence for these is not conclusive.

Conception should be possible, then, only when sexual relations take place just around the time of ovulation. At other times, intercourse presumably cannot lead to a pregnancy, because there is not a viable egg present and because sperm will not live long enough to wait for the subsequent egg. This is the basis for the theory that there is a safe period in the menstrual cycle, and for the rhythm method of birth control.

Then to tell when the safe period is, it would be necessary first to know when ovulation takes place.

Exactly. However, at present it is impossible to pinpoint with certainty the exact time in the menstrual cycle when this happens. All we know for certain is that ovulation occurs approximately twelve to sixteen days before the beginning of a menses.

Are there any physical manifestations at the time of ovulation—any recognizable symptoms?

Well, there are changes in the secretion found at the opening of the uterus and in the cells found in the vagina, but it would of course require laboratory analysis to detect them.

As I told you earlier, some women do report a sensation of discomfort or even pain in the lower part of the abdomen, or a low backache, during ovulation time, and this may be accompanied by slight vaginal spotting. If these symptoms occur regularly on a certain day of the menstrual cycle, they probably signify that the woman is either ovulating or is about to ovulate at that time. Such phenomena occur, though, in only a small percentage of women, and most women are quite unaware of the time of their ovulation.

Is there any way, then, of telling in advance when ovulation will take place?

Unfortunately, there is no way of predicting the exact day when ovulation will occur. Available methods tell us only the probable day when ovulation *has occurred*. There are some indirect signs of impending ovulation, such as changes in the secretion found at the opening of the uterus and in the cells found in the vagina, but the most popular way of telling when ovulation has occurred is to keep a careful record of the menstrual periods for about eight to twelve months. Such a record may, in itself, sometimes be sufficient to indicate fairly accurately the probable day of ovulation. Normally the egg is released from the ovary twelve to sixteen days before the onset of the next menstruation. If the length and variations of a woman's menstrual cycle are known, then it may be possible to calculate the probable day of ovulation.

Just what is the menstrual cycle?

The menstrual cycle is the interval between the beginning of one menstruation and the beginning of the next. The day on which the flow first appears is counted as the first day, or day number one, of the cycle, and the day before the next flow begins as the last day.

The Time of Ovulation

How does a woman calculate the probable time of ovulation?

As I said, ovulation occurs twelve to sixteen days before the beginning of the next menses. If a woman menstruates regularly every twenty-eight days, then her ovulation will take place between the thirteenth and seventeenth day of her cycle, counting from the first day on which her menstruation began. If the cycles are shorter, the day of ovulation will come earlier; if longer, ovulation will occur later. In other words, the number of days between the beginning of menstruation and the time of ovulation may vary considerably, but the number of days between ovulation and the beginning of the following menstruation is usually fairly constant.

Does a woman usually have her menstrual periods at regular intervals?

No, as a rule the cycles are somewhat irregular. While the average menstrual cycle is about twenty-eight days, there is usually a fluctuation of several days between one cycle and another in the same woman; some cycles are shorter and some longer. Variations in normal cycles may go from twenty-one to thirty-five days. Generally, however, the difference between a woman's shortest and longest cycles in a year is not more than about six to eight days.

If the periods are irregular, is it still possible to calculate the time of ovulation from the menstrual record?

If the variations between cycles are not too great, the probable time of ovulation can still be estimated. Suppose that a study of the menstrual calendar shows that during the year the cycles had varied from twenty-six to thirty-two days. If the woman's menstrual period, let us say, now begins on the first of August, then her next menstrual period would presumably come not earlier than the twenty-seventh of August and not later than the second of September. If we then consider that ovulation occurs about 12 to 16 days before the onset of the next period, in this case it could come on any day between the eleventh and the twenty-first of August. This is the closest that the ovulation day can be calculated on the basis of the menstrual record.

Calculation of the "Safe Period"

Now, supposing that a woman keeps a careful calendar record of her periods, how is the actual safe period calculated?

If the record shows that a woman menstruates regularly every twenty-eight days, then she presumably ovulates between the thirteenth and the seventeenth day, counting from the first day of her preceding menstruation. However, since the sperm may remain alive for several days, and we do not know for how long the egg may be fertilizable, extra days are added for safety.

The fertile period is calculated by subtracting eleven from the longest recorded cycle and eighteen from the shortest cycle. The fertile period, therefore, which means the days of abstinence, will extend between and including those two days. And the *safe period* will include all the other days of the cycle.

Let us suppose that a woman's cycles have varied during the preceding year from twenty-five to thirty-three days. Her fertile period can be calculated by subtracting eighteen from twenty-five (25 − 18 = 7), and subtracting eleven from thirty-three (33 − 11 = 22); it extends therefore from day number seven to day number twenty-two inclusive, and sexual abstinence should be observed all through those days.

Could a woman herself calculate her safe period on the basis of her menstrual record?

Yes. As we said before, if a careful record of the menstrual cycles has been kept, it is very possible for a woman to do it correctly. However, since the risk of unplanned pregnancy may cause so much mental strain, it may be advisable for her to consult with a person competent and experienced in this method.

A great variety of calculating devices and gadgets are advertised to aid in this calculation. However, these are not always reliable, and they do not ease the task, since a record of the menstrual cycle must still be kept.

Unanticipated physical or psychological factors sometimes unexpectedly change a woman's menstrual rhythm, and with it also the time of the safe period. Anxiety, illness, or unusual excitement such as a vacation or moving may change the length of the menstrual cycle; the safe-period method will be less reliable as long as the unusual conditions last.

How reliable is the rhythm method?

If rhythm is practiced according to the method which we have just discussed—that is, the "calendar method"—it may be as reliable as some of the chemical contraceptive methods.

The Temperature Method

Is it possible to make the rhythm method safer?

Yes, by keeping another kind of record. After ovulation, the temperature of the body goes up slightly and stays up until the start of the next menstrual period. This sustained rise in temperature is an indication that ovulation has already taken place. The change can be observed only if the temperature is taken immediately on waking, every day, before rising, smoking, or even drinking water. At that time the temperature is at its lowest and represents what is called the "basal body temperature."

If taken regularly during an entire cycle, either by mouth or, preferably, rectally, the basal body temperature shows a characteristic curve. During the first part of the cycle it is at its lowest, ranging from about ninety-seven to ninety-eight degrees Fahrenheit, but rarely going above ninety-eight degrees. The temperature curve then shows a distinct rise over a period of one to three days. Thereafter it stays at a higher level, usually about ninety-eight to ninety-nine degrees, for the remaining days of the cycle until near the onset of menses. The shift in temperature from the low to the high corresponds closely to the time of ovulation.

If a woman, therefore, wishes to determine the approximate day of ovulation, she may do so by taking her temperature as soon as she awakens and recording it on a special chart for a period of one or two months. Her physician can then show her how to tell the ovulation day by means of the chart.

Can the temperature record, then, be used to determine the safe period?

Since the rise in temperature is a signal that ovulation has already taken place, this method cannot be used to determine the first fertile day, but it may make it possible to resume intercourse a few days earlier than otherwise.

Sexual relations should be avoided from the first fertile day (computed by subtracting eighteen from the shortest menstrual cycle recorded during the preceding year) until the evening of the third day after the temperature rise, when they can be safely resumed. Since a slight cold or a stomach upset may affect the body temperature, this guide must be used with considerable caution.

Couples wishing to have no more pregnancies should rely only on the temperature record—that is, observe sexual abstinence from menses until the temperature has risen and remained high for three consecutive days, and limit intercourse to the remainder of the cycle. The efficacy of the rhythm method, if strictly used in this way, can be equal or superior to that of any of the mechanical or chemical methods or of the intra-uterine devices.

At times the temperature record may be quite irregular and rather confusing to one with little experience in interpreting the chart. If a woman wishes to rely on the temperature cycle as a birth-control method, it is best to obtain the advice of an experienced physician. After a while she may learn to read the chart herself.

Evaluation of the "Safe Period"

What is your opinion of the safe period as a contraceptive method?

Well, if a woman's menstrual periods are not too irregular, or if she keeps an accurate temperature record, it may be possible for the physician to calculate with considerable certainty the days of the month when she will be safe from conception. If her cycles fluctuate too widely, then such calculations are difficult to make and are not reliable.

From the point of view of fertility, the menstrual month can be divided into three periods: the infertile days before ovulation, the fertile days around ovulation time, and again the infertile days after ovulation has taken place. Of the two safe periods during the cycle, the first, or the preovulatory, is the less certain, because we do not yet know exactly how long the sperm may retain their vitality within the genital tract of the woman. The second part of the safe period, the postovulatory, is the more reliable, because by that time there is no possibility of an egg's being released or of a viable egg's being present to be fertilized.

For practical purposes, if we divide the menstrual month into three equal parts, the first third is comparatively safe, the middle third is the fertile time, and the last third is, as far as our present knowledge is concerned, quite safe from conception. Thus, if a woman, for instance, menstruates every thirty days, she would be comparatively safe during the first ten days; she would be fertile during the second ten days; and she would be quite free from the possibility of conception during the last ten days. However, it is not advisable to rely on such rough approximations.

Do failures ever occur when this method is followed?

Yes, failures do occur not infrequently among women who rely exclusively on the calendar method of calculating the safe period. In most instances these failures are no doubt due to careless or inaccurate calculations or recordings. In some cases, however, the failures result from some physical or emotional condition which unexpectedly alters the length of the cycle and the day of ovulation. It is well established that ailments of one kind or another, as well as marked anxieties and emotional tensions, may disturb the regularity of the reproductive cycle, making it either shorter or longer, and thus changing the day of ovulation and hence of the safe period.

However, it is possible to make rhythm a very effective birth-control method by relying exclusively on the basal-body-temperature record. As we said before, if rhythm is used strictly following the temperature record, it can be almost as effective as any other method available today.

Aside from its safety, doesn't reliance on the safe period interfere with the normal rhythm of sexual desire?

From a psychosexual viewpoint reliance on the safe period has certain drawbacks. In many animal species the female will generally accept the male only during her fertile period, but reliance on the safe period involves complete abstinence during the time of the month when the woman is most fertile, at the time when there may be considerable sexual interest on her part. From this viewpoint, the safe period is certainly not a "natural" method.

Many women, however, use the safe period as an additional or alternative method of contraception, rather than as the sole one.

They resort to contraceptives during the fertile days and then rely only upon the safe period during the days when the chances of a conception are at a minimum. The fact that unprotected intercourse is thus made possible during at least a third of the month is welcomed by many couples.

Some years ago we established a special safe-period service at the Margaret Sanger Research Bureau, where the individual safe period is calculated for women who bring in a record of their menstrual cycles covering the preceding ten or twelve months. Many of these women continue to use contraceptives during their fertile days, but discontinue them during the safe days, and find this plan very satisfactory.

Is it not surprising that after so many centuries man should still be in doubt about the time or the reliability of the safe period?

Yes, this again shows how recent is most of our knowledge about human reproduction. It is highly encouraging, however, that the social and biological aspects of human fertility are being studied more actively today than ever before. There can be little doubt that in the decades to come many significant advances will be made in our knowledge of the human reproductive cycle.

Isn't there a chemical test for detecting ovulation?

A rat test was developed by Dr. Farris for the detection of ovulation, and in his hands it proved to be very reliable. However, it is expensive and impractical to repeat every month, and many investigators have been unable to obtain the same results.

Chemical or color tests, made by placing a piece of paper tape in the vagina, have also been described from time to time. However, all the investigations of these tests conducted at the Margaret Sanger Research Bureau have proved them to be quite unreliable. A new color test, based on the salt contents of the secretion found at the opening of the uterus, is being presently investigated, and the results obtained are more encouraging.

What other methods are available for the prevention of conception?

In a general way, contraceptive methods can be divided into "male methods," or those that can be used by the husband, and "female methods," or those that can be used by the wife. I want to emphasize again, however, that the choice of a contraceptive should be made individually in consultation with a physician.

Male Methods

If the husband wishes to take the precautions, what methods can he use?

For the man there are only two methods available. Both of them have the purpose of preventing the seminal fluid from entering the vaginal canal during intercourse.

One of the methods has a rather venerable history. It is described, in fact, in some detail in the Bible, in connection with the story of Onan, although it was undoubtedly resorted to long before Biblical times, perhaps ever since man realized the relation between sex union and conception.

Coitus Interruptus

What is the story of Onan? I remember having read it in the Bible, but I can't recall the details now.

There was an ancient Hebrew law or custom that when a married man died without leaving a son, his unmarried brother, if he had one, was required to marry the widow, and the firstborn son of this union was to be named after the deceased brother. A young man by the name of Onan found himself in such a situation; his elder brother had been killed, and it was now his duty to marry the widow. For one reason or another, however, Onan did not want to bring up children in his brother's name, and so, as the story in Genesis reads: "When he went in unto his brother's wife . . . he spilled it on the ground, lest he should give seed to his brother." In other words, Onan resorted to a method of preventing conception, a method which is practiced very widely even today—namely, withdrawal, or, as it is technically known, coitus interruptus. The male organ is withdrawn just prior to the ejaculation, and the seminal fluid is discharged outside the female genital tract.

Did the term "onanism" arise from this story? I always thought that onanism referred to masturbation.

This is a rather common impression, and the term is even so defined in some dictionaries. From the Biblical story, however, it seems clear that Onan resorted not to masturbation but to withdrawal before completion of the sex act, in order to prevent conception and avoid bringing up a child in his brother's name.

Is withdrawal a satisfactory method?

Aside from abortion and infanticide, withdrawal is the oldest birth-control method in practice. Probably the reduction in the number of births in most of the developed countries was accomplished through this method before modern birth-control methods became available. It has been heavily criticized, and you may have heard or read statements condemning it as unreliable, unsatisfactory, and even physiologically and psychologically unsound. The only truth that the criticisms may have is that this method is not fully reliable, since in the excitement of the sexual act it is sometimes difficult for the man to withdraw in time so that not a single drop of his semen is deposited in the vagina of the woman.

If the man is able to control his orgasm until his wife has reached hers, the method can be fully satisfactory to both partners. In any case, this convenient and inexpensive method should not be overlooked, for the occasion may occur in which the temporary unavailability of other contraceptive measures may expose the couple to unwelcome risks. At such a time withdrawal may be a useful technique.

Coitus Reservatus

What is coitus reservatus? Is it a method of birth control?

Yes, it is a practice somewhat similar to withdrawal, or coitus interruptus; but it differs from withdrawal in that the man abstains completely from ejaculation during intercourse. This method of conception control was practiced by the members of the Oneida Community about a century ago.

Do you mean that the husband does not ejaculate at all?

Yes. According to what is reported in the Oneida group, the men, by training themselves, were able to continue the act of coitus with many intermissions for one or two hours or even longer without reaching a climax. This practice was resorted to partly as a contraceptive measure and partly under the belief that the retention of the seminal fluid was of some particular benefit to the man. However, there is no scientific basis whatsoever for this theory.

The Sheath
What other methods can a man use?

A much more practical male method to prevent the sperm from entering the vagina is the use of a cover which is placed over the male organ during intercourse. This cover, commonly known as the male sheath or the condom, was first suggested some four hundred years ago. The sheath really serves a twofold purpose: by retaining the seminal discharge it prevents conception, and by covering the penis may prevent the transmission of venereal infections. It must be remembered that as a method for the prevention of venereal diseases, it is a poor and unreliable one.

There are two main types of sheath: the so-called "skin" made of a special animal tissue, and the rubber sheaths which are prepared from latex rubber. The skins are available premoistened, and they should not be allowed to dry before use; they are generally more expensive and have no special advantage over those made of latex. Latex condoms are made with either a blunt or a teat end, and can be obtained either lubricated or plain.

What is your opinion of the condom? Is it a reliable method?

If the condom is fresh and of good quality, and if it is used properly, it is unquestionably a very reliable method of birth control.

What is the proper way to use a condom?

This is a very good question, because many people regard this method as so simple that no instructions are needed. However, a few precautions should be mentioned. It is good always to apply the condom to the penis when it is in full erection but before it has made any contact with the genitals of the woman. It is also advisable, in the case of an uncircumcised man, for the foreskin to be fully retracted. A portion of the tip of the condom, about an inch, should be left free at the tip of the penis; this portion should also be free of air, allowing room for intromission and the sexual movements to occur without unduly stretching the rubber. It also provides room for the ejaculate and thus prevents it from leaking out.

On the completion of intercourse, and before the penis has lost its erection, the condom should be grasped against the base of the penis and withdrawn in such a way as not to spill a single drop of semen.

Should a condom be tested before use?

In the United States, condoms are individually tested before packing. If the condom is fresh and of a reputable brand bought in a drugstore, testing by the user is unnecessary and would probably only weaken the rubber. However, in the event that the quality of the condom is questionable, the simplest way of testing is to unroll it and blow it up with a single puff to not more than two inches in diameter and hold it in front of a light.

To decrease the chances of a condom breaking, as well as to avoid irritation, sufficient lubrication should be present. If natural moisture is absent, an artificial lubricant, preferably one of the so-called contraceptive jellies, should be applied to the outside of the condom after it is adjusted, and some men prefer to use a little of the lubricant on the inside of the condom as well. The cover should not be applied too tightly (leaving, as I said before, about one inch free and empty of air) over the head or glans of the penis. If there is uncertainty as to the quality of the condom it may be advisable to have a douche available in the event that the condom should break during use.

Is the use of the condom in any way injurious? Can it cause any harm to the man or to the woman?

No, as far as we know the condom does not produce any harmful effects, and many people find this method quite satisfactory. It certainly can be classed among the better methods available for contraceptive purposes. Some women, it is true, experience some local irritation when it is used, but this can be obviated to a large degree by proper lubrication. A more serious objection perhaps is the fact that it has to be applied after the erection has already been attained and hence necessitates an interruption of sexual foreplay. In some cases this proves to be psychologically disturbing to the man and affects his sexual capacity and response. If his potency is inadequate, it may add considerably to the difficulty. However, for couples not unusually shy and who approach sexual relations with full freedom and spontaneous cooperation, the placement of the condom on the male organ can be made a very satisfactory part of the precoital sexual play. The condom also prevents direct contact of the penis with the vagina during the sex relation and thus tends to diminish sensation for the man. However, this may prove to be an advantage for men who have a tendency to early ejaculation, since it may enable them to prolong intercourse and thus provide more enjoyment for both partners.

Female Methods

What kinds of birth-control methods can a woman use?

A woman has many more choices of contraceptives than the man, whose methods, as we have just seen, can be directed to only one aim—preventing the entry of the seminal fluid into the vagina.

When sperm are deposited in the vagina during intercourse, in order for conception to take place they must pass into the uterus and through the uterus into the tubes, where they meet the egg. Female methods of preventing conception work in varied ways and at various stages of this reproductive process. Many of the methods are designed to keep the sperm from going any farther than the vagina. Until the mid-1950s virtually all available female methods—some of them chemical, some mechanical and others a combination of the two—had this object, and some of these are still highly regarded. Later developments are the mechanical devices which function in the uterus rather than in the vagina, and which prevent pregnancy by an action not yet entirely understood; and the oral contraceptives which stop ovulation temporarily.

The Douche

A still widely used method is the douche, which is designed to remove the seminal fluid from the vagina after intercourse. If all the sperm can be removed or destroyed by the douche before they have a chance to get into the uterus, conception will not occur. The addition of antiseptics to the douche presumably enhances its protective value by destroying the sperm, but plain water, or water and vinegar (a tablespoon of vinegar to a quart of water), is probably as effective for this purpose as any of the commercially advertised antiseptics. While some women use the douches satisfactorily for long periods of time, the percentage of failures with this method is high, and it should not be relied upon as the sole measure of protection.

How soon after intercourse should a douche for preventive purposes be taken?

You will recall that though the sperm travel at the rate of about an inch in eight minutes or so, they can enter the opening of the womb almost immediately after ejaculation. Hence, even if they have not entered the uterus during intercourse they may reach the uterine canal within a very few minutes. In order, therefore, to be at all effective, the douche should be taken as soon after sexual contact as possible, preferably within five minutes.

What is the best way of taking a douche?

The sitting position, on the toilet, is the most convenient. The douche bag should be hung so that its bottom is no higher than the top of the woman's head when she is seated. This supplies sufficient pressure for the purpose. The nozzle should be inserted for about three inches, depending upon the depth of the vagina. While the water is flowing in, the woman should contract the muscles around the vaginal outlet, or else compress the labia with her fingers, relaxing the muscles and opening the canal at intervals to permit the water to flow out. In this manner the canal is well distended and a thorough flushing is obtained.

Are some kinds of devices for douching purposes better than others?

There are two general kinds of douching appliances: the usual rubber bag and the hand-bulb syringe. The nozzles too vary in length, thickness and shape. The ordinary bag-and-nozzle is probably just as satisfactory as any of the more complicated types, and certainly less apt to produce injury.

Is the use of a douche alone sufficient to prevent conception?

No, I should say that the douche alone is not a reliable measure. You will remember that it is possible for the sperm to enter the uterus very soon after the ejaculation. It is even maintained by some that at the end of the sexual act the female uterus exerts an actual suction, so that a certain amount of the seminal fluid is drawn into it directly, though no modern investigator has been able to prove this. At any rate, the douche can remove only the fluid which is in the vagina; it will not affect the sperm cells that have already entered the cervix. Furthermore, you will recall that the vaginal walls are not smooth but have numerous small folds. Unless the vagina is thoroughly distended and cleansed during douching there is some possibility that a little of the seminal fluid may remain in these folds and not be affected by the solution employed.

Aside from the fact that the douche is not sufficiently reliable, the necessity for arising immediately after intercourse is also a serious objection to its use as a contraceptive method. As we shall see later, it is desirable that a certain period of rest and relaxation should follow the sexual relation, and this rest is disturbed if the woman has to douche immediately after contact. The chief value of the douche, then, is either as an auxiliary to other methods or as an emergency method when needed.

Chemical Contraceptives

If a chemical contraceptive is to be relied upon, it should be of the type that is to be placed in the vagina prior to rather than after the sex act. Products available for this purpose are made up in the form of suppositories, tablets, powders, jellies or creams, and they consist of various bases into which certain chemical ingredients are incorporated. In the vaginal canal these preparations dissolve or spread along the vaginal walls and over the uterine opening, forming a mechanical barrier to the passage of the sperm. At the same time the liberated chemical ingredients are intended to immobilize the sperm and render them inactive.

Suppositories

Are suppositories reliable, Doctor? I have seen them advertised as effective for feminine hygiene.

Suppositories are made by incorporating one or more chemical ingredients in a cocoa-butter, gelatine or other base which is solid under normal temperatures but melts at body heat. When introduced into the vagina, the suppository is supposed to dissolve and thus to liberate its chemical contents. It is assumed that the base, after melting, will form an oily or gelatinous layer over the mouth of the uterus, producing a mechanical barrier to the entrance of the sperm, while the chemicals will serve to immobilize them. To be effective, therefore, the suppositiory must melt readily, but this does not always occur. At times we have found suppositories unmelted in the vagina even half an hour after insertion. Even if the suppository does melt, it may not cover the uterine opening, and, since it appears to be possible for the sperm to enter the uterus very soon after coitus, it is obvious that the suppositories will have no effect under such circumstances. There is always, therefore, a strong element of chance in relying on suppositories for protection. Many people also object to them because of the excessive oiliness or greasiness which is produced when they melt.

"Feminine hygiene" is frequently merely a euphemism for contraception, and all kinds of products are extravagantly advertised for that purpose. It is unfortunate indeed that some commercial concerns make inaccurate and misleading claims in matters that involve the health and welfare of people.

It is possible that a thoroughly reliable and acceptable suppository may eventually be developed, but for the present none that I know are entirely dependable.

Vaginal Tablets and Powders

Somewhat similar drawbacks apply to the chemical contraceptives put up in the form of foam tablets. The tablets, on dissolving in the vagina, liberate a gas which forms a foam in the vagina and acts as both a chemical and a mechanical contraceptive. In order for the tablet to dissolve, however, a certain amount of moisture is required, and sometimes the moisture normally present in the vagina is insufficient. Occasionally we have found tablets in the vagina undissolved after half an hour. Or if they do dissolve, the foam may disappear so quickly that it can hardly have any effect.

Jellies and Creams

What about jellies and creams? Are they more reliable?

Of the several chemical contraceptives available, the jellies and creams are, I believe, the most adequate. Because they are already in a semisolid or creamy state they do not have to melt or dissolve in order to be effective, and on account of their consistency they spread much more readily along the vaginal canal and across the uterine opening. They are put up in collapsible tubes. Special syringe-like applicators are available by which a measured amount of the jelly, cream or foam can be introduced into the vagina. Jellies, however, sometimes cause overlubrication or leakage from the vagina, and this is an aesthetic drawback to their use. Newer products are constantly being developed and some of them are highly effective.

Is there any danger that chemical contraceptives might be injurious in some way?

The chemical contraceptives are not apt to be injurious. Should the ingredients of a particular product be too strong or too concentrated, or should a woman happen to be particularly sensitive to any of the chemicals employed, there is a possibility of some irritation to the tissues. In an examination of a very large number of women, however, we have seen but very few instances of local irritation that could be ascribed to the use of chemical contraceptives. It is important, nevertheless, that the ingredients employed in contraceptives be harmless, and that for douching purposes strong solutions be avoided.

Both contraceptive jellies, creams and foam creams are now available to provide contraceptive protection without being irritating to the delicate tissues of the genital tract. In addition, foam creams are available without prescription; these, like some of the creams and jellies, have been exhaustively tested in both the laboratory and the Contraception Service of the Margaret Sanger Research Bureau, and have been found highly acceptable and effective. However, their effectiveness does not reach that of the condom, the diaphragm or the intra-uterine device, much less that of the contraceptive pills, which are virtually 100 per cent effective.

Mechanical Contraceptives

Far more reliable are the mechanical contraceptives—mainly the vaginal diaphragm, which covers up the entrance to the uterus and forms a mechanical barrier to the passage of the sperm from the vagina into the cervix, and the various intra-uterine devices.

Vaginal Diaphragms

The diaphragm, also called the pessary, was introduced to this country by Margaret Sanger and popularized among the thousands of women who flocked to her birth-control clinic, and it is still considered one of the most effective contraceptive methods ever devised. Designed to lie diagonally across the vaginal canal, covering the cervix, it comes in a large variety of shapes and sizes. Usually it consists of a dome of soft rubber or latex, from two to four inches in diameter, with a thick elastic metal rim. It is not possible to tell the size that a woman requires without gynecological examination. Since considerable variations exist in pelvic anatomy, a woman should no more use a diaphragm which has not been fitted for her individually than she should use a pair of eyeglasses which have not been prescribed for her particular needs.

Is it difficult to learn how to use a diaphragm?

It requires some minimal manual dexterity, which can be acquired with a bit of practice. If the woman is fitted with the diaphragm by a physician competent in the prescription of this method and follows his instructions, she should have little or no difficulty.

Before inserting the diaphragm, she applies about a teaspoon of contraceptive cream or jelly to the inside of the dome and around the rim; this acts as a lubricant to make insertion easier, and as an additional contraceptive safeguard. She then introduces the diaphragm into the vagina either manually or with the aid of a special inserter. When it has slipped into place, she inserts a finger to make sure that the cervix is covered and to place the anterior part of the rim behind the pubic bone out front.

At the Sanger Bureau, where some forty per cent of the clients still prefer the diaphragm to the several other methods offered to them, each woman who is fitted with the device is given detailed instructions on how to use it and is told to practice at home for a week or so, then to return and demonstrate her ability to perform the diaphragm insertion and removal correctly. Most women who faithfully follow this procedure master the technique with little difficulty and can thereafter rely upon the diaphragm with confidence for contraceptive protection.

When should the diaphragm be inserted and for how long should it be left in?

It may be inserted either before retiring or immediately before the sexual relation. Unlike the intra-uterine devices, which we will discuss later, the diaphragm, or pessary, cannot be left in place indefinitely, but should be removed within twenty-four hours and be inserted anew when the couple are again to have sexual relations. Exactly how long it is to remain in place after intercourse depends entirely upon the convenience of the woman. If she wishes, she may remove it immediately, or else she may leave it in until the next day. If she does remove it soon after coitus, however, she should douche both before and after removal in order to wash out the seminal fluid from the canal. For this purpose, plain warm water is sufficient and as effective as any of the commercially advertised solutions.

But didn't you say before, Doctor, that the douche is unreliable because it does not always prevent the sperm from entering the womb?

Yes, but that applies only when the douche is the sole method of protection. With the pessary in place, the sperm cannot go up into the uterus during intercourse, and the fluid remaining in the canal can then be washed out quite thoroughly.

Is a douche necessary if the diaphragm is left in place until the next morning?

No. In a number of examinations we have found that with the diaphragm in place there were no active sperm in the vagina three to four hours after sexual contact, and it is quite likely that they lose their vitality even sooner. Hence, if the diaphragm is permitted to remain in place that length of time, it may be removed without a preliminary douche.

Once a woman has been fitted with a diaphragm, does it have to be refitted often?

The doctor may ask the woman to return for a checkup examination within a week to make certain that she inserts the diaphragm correctly. Thereafter an annual examination is quite sufficient. The diaphragm should also be examined frequently to make sure it is in good condition and has not been damaged. With ordinary care, it should last from one to two years or even longer. After childbirth or after a gynecological operation, a reexamination is essential, for the anatomical changes that take place during childbearing and childbirth or after operative procedures often necessitate a different type or size of diaphragm.

Do you consider the diaphragm to be a reliable contraceptive?

Yes, it is both reliable and satisfactory. The diaphragm covers the opening of the uterus and thus prevents the entry of the sperm; at the same time it permits direct contact between the male organ and the vaginal wall, so that sensation is little affected. If the correct size is chosen, neither the woman nor the man should be conscious of its presence. Furthermore, it can be inserted long before use so that the normal sequence of the sexual act need not be disturbed.

Is the diaphragm a suitable method for all women?

No. First of all, the diaphragm cannot be prescribed while the hymen is still intact. For the first two or three weeks of marriage, therefore, it is the man who must employ preventive measures if a conception is to be avoided, unless the hymen is artificially dilated by a physician before marriage. Then too some women cannot be fitted with a diaphragm because of variations in anatomical structure of the genital tract. The muscular relaxations which sometimes follow difficult childbirths, for instance, may make the diaphragm unsuitable, and other protective devices will then have to be employed.

Cervical Caps

Are there other mechanical methods that can be used when a diaphragm is not suitable?

When a diaphragm cannot be used, a cervical cap is sometimes prescribed. The cap is designed to be placed directly over the opening of the uterus, the cervix, over which it fits snugly. Cervical caps are usually made of plastic, though they may also be of rubber, and they come in several sizes. After the physician has chosen the correct size, the woman is taught how to insert and remove the cap herself. She uses it just as she would a diaphragm, inserting it when needed and leaving it in place until the next morning.

Intra-uterine Devices

Can you tell us about the intra-uterine devices?

Intra-uterine contraception has been used from time immemorial. Arabs are said to insert small stones into the uterus of their female camels to prevent them from getting pregnant while on long trips through the desert. This type of contraception was also used in women at the end of the last century and in the early part of this century. It was heavily criticized, since it produced a lot of undesirable effects, such as bleeding and infection, and it was virtually abandoned, except by a few Japanese and European gynecologists.

In 1959 two important papers appeared in the medical literature, one by Dr. Ishihama of Japan, the other by Dr. Oppenheimer, a German immigrant in Israel. These two doctors reported the satisfactory use of intra-uterine contraceptive devices in large numbers of women for many years. Their reports aroused a new interest, and many gynecologists started to work on the idea of a device to be inserted into the uterus and left there indefinitely, being removed only when its contraceptive protection was no longer desired.

How do these devices work?

A great deal of speculation, not all of it scientific, is still going on as to how the device can provide contraceptive protection, and some have gone so far as to say that it does so by producing abortions when the egg is too small for a pregnancy to be detected.

Available scientific information indicates that the devices work in many different ways, depending on the animal species studied. Presently, it is impossible to state clearly how they work in humans. It seems quite possible, however, that the transit of the egg through the Fallopian tube is speeded up to such an extent that fertilization becomes impossible.

What are these devices like?

Many different shapes have been designed by gynecologists interested in this type of contraception. Ota in Japan uses a device made of polyethylene that looks very much like a wheel with three curving spokes. Dr. Oppenheimer used one ring made of several turns of silkworm gut. Dr. Zipper of Chile uses a nylon fishing filament coiled in the shape of a ring. In the United States Dr. Hall designed a flexible ring made of a fine spiral coil of stainless-steel wire, but all other devices used in this country are made of polyethylene plastic, which is apparently well tolerated by the human body and also very inexpensive. The two most used in the United States are the Lippes "loop" and the Margulies "spiral." The Lippes loop is a polyethylene rod in the shape of a double S, and the Margulies spiral is a rod in the shape of a flattened coil. There are other devices, like the intra-uterine "bow" designed by Dr. Birnberg in the shape of two triangles joined at the apex, and a new device, the Majzlin spring, a flattened spring made of very elastic stainless steel.

How are they put into the uterus?

They must be inserted by a doctor who is familiar with this type of contraception. The loop or the spiral can be compressed and put into a narrow plastic tube resembling a soda straw, which is then placed into the opening of the womb. With the help of a plunger the device is pushed from the tube into the womb, where it resumes its original shape, and the tube is withdrawn.

The stainless-steel ring and the plastic bow are also made as narrow as possible, and are inserted in a similar manner into the womb.

Is it painful to have this done?

Some discomfort or even mild pain is always involved in the insertion of an intra-uterine device. Sometimes it may even be necessary to slightly dilate the opening of the womb to make insertion possible. The discomfort, however, does not last very long; it usually disappears the same day. It is usually compared to menstrual cramps, and in general a few aspirin tablets or similar painkiller will be enough to control it.

Since the opening of the womb is wider at the time of menstruation, and since insertion may be accompanied by some staining or bleeding, many doctors favor inserting the device during the menstrual period.

Can any woman use these devices?

Intra-uterine devices are advised almost exclusively for women who already have had children. The enlarged opening of the womb makes insertion easier, and the uterine walls, which have already been stretched, tolerate better the presence of the device.

What happens when she wants to have a baby?

All of the devices can be easily removed by the doctor. Some of them, like the loop and the spiral and the spring, are provided with a "tail" by which they are simply pulled out; for the other devices, such as the ring or the bow, a special instrument must be used.

After removal of the device, normal fertility is immediately resumed.

Is the removal painful?

Some discomfort may accompany the removal of the intra-uterine device, but not in all cases. Removal is less painful than insertion, and if there is pain it passes quickly.

How long can the device be left in the womb? Must it be removed for cleaning?

The devices are made of an inert material which is not affected by body secretions, so it is not necessary to remove them for cleaning. They may be left in place indefinitely, for as long as contraception is necessary or desired.

Are there any problems connected with the use of these devices?

The most common problem in the use of intra-uterine devices is persistent pain or bleeding, or both. Some women may find that the mild discomfort and staining that accompany insertion fail to disappear or even that they get worse. If the pain is too intense to be mitigated by common analgesics such as aspirin, or if the bleeding is too profuse or lasts too long, the doctor may advise removal of the device.

Another problem frequently encountered is that the uterus may contract and expel the device, especially during a menstrual period. For this reason, menstrual pads or tampons should always be inspected when removed; and after menses, if the device has a "tail," the woman should insert a clean finger into her vagina and feel for the tail in order to assure herself that the device is still in place.

Is it possible for pregnancy to occur if a device is in place?

Despite the many interesting and serious scientific studies made, we do not know as yet how the intra-uterine contraceptive devices work in the human. We do know that except for the Pill the intra-uterine device is the most effective contraceptive method presently available. However, some unintended pregnancies do occur even while the device is in place. With the most successful devices, approximately two to three pregnancies may occur in one hundred women during the first year of use; the rate is lower after the first year. Of such accidental pregnancies, two out of three occur with the device in place, the others in women who have failed to notice a spontaneous expulsion of the device.

Although many will regard with concern such a possibility of accidental pregnancy, this rate compares favorably with those of many other available contraceptive methods. It should also be recognized that before the oral pills—which not all women can or want to take—the amount of protection afforded by the intra-uterine devices would have seemed fully satisfactory to both users and doctors.

What should be done with the device if pregnancy occurs while it is still in place? Can it be taken out?

There is no danger to either the mother or the baby if the device is left in the womb. The device will be outside the bag of waters and will not interfere at all with the pregnancy. Most doctors prefer not to touch the device after a pregnancy has occurred, since the device is sometimes expelled spontaneously by the pregnant uterus and certainly after the delivery—most likely together with the afterbirth.

Are intra-uterine devices harmful? I have heard that they may cause cancer.

As we mentioned, modern intra-uterine devices are made of inert materials which are nonirritating to the tissues. Furthermore, the lining of the womb renews itself every month, when menstruation occurs, and the tissues in contact with the device change at this time.

In the United States, extensive experience has shown that thus far there is no reason to believe that the continued presence of such a device will induce the development of cancer. It may be reassuring to remember that foreign bodies are left sometimes within a person's body for his entire life without any harmful effect. I am referring to the sutures and knots used by the surgeon, to plastic replacements of sections of arteries or veins, to stainless-steel pins or plates in bones, and to permanent dental replacements.

Non-prescription Methods of Birth Control

What could people do about birth control if they lived far away from a doctor or a clinic or a family-planning center?

Well, we have already mentioned several methods that are available without prescription. If there is a drugstore where condoms, foam creams or jellies and creams designed for use without a diaphragm are available, one of these may meet the need. Or the drugstore may be able to supply spermicidal vaginal suppositories or foaming tablets.

An older and still less expensive device is a small sponge moistened with a lather-producing liquid, or with water and a lather-producing powder, or with a salt solution. Modern latex foam sponges, small sea sponges or little powder puffs—about the size of a hen's egg—are excellent for this purpose; a string may be attached through the center to facilitate removal. Small wads of cloth or other soft fiber have also been used.

The vaginal douche (which, you should remember, has virtually no value as a contraceptive unless used immediately after ejaculation has occurred) is a somewhat more sophisticated method and requires a toilet or some other outlet for the water in the douche bag, but the other methods mentioned above can all be used without benefit of plumbing, and even with a minimum of privacy.

While all these methods are less effective than more modern ones, they are nevertheless a great deal more useful than no method at all.

The Pill

Will you tell us about "the Pill"?

In the mid-1950s scientists found a way to produce a number of synthetic substances which can be easily and cheaply manufactured and which, when taken by mouth in very small dosages, have an effect similar to that of the hormones produced normally by a woman's ovaries. In certain combinations these synthetic hormones—called estrogens and progestagens—can be used to suppress ovulation or to regulate the menstrual cycle, or both. It is these hormones that make "the Pill" the most effective contraceptive yet devised, when properly taken under medical supervision.

How do these hormones work?

We have already discussed the direct relationship that exists between the ovaries and the pituitary gland at the base of the brain. The pituitary gland, through stimulus received from the nearby base of the brain (the hypothalamus), produces a number of stimulating hormones, some of which direct the normal functioning of the ovaries and are called gonadotropins. These hormones are also produced in men and are responsible for the functioning of the testes. In women, the gonadotropins act upon the ovaries, causing some of the ovarian follicles—where the eggs nest—to develop and to produce estrogens. When one of the follicles matures and releases an egg, estrogens and progesterone are carried into the bloodstream of the woman. There these ovarian hormones act on certain centers in the base of the brain and slow down the production of pituitary hormones. As the pituitary hormones diminish, the production of hormones by the ovaries is also diminished. Then the braking action of the ovarian hormones upon the pituitary gland disappears, and the gland is again able to start producing its own stimulating hormones, which in turn stimulate the ovaries and their follicles to develop; ovulation occurs, and the whole cycle starts again.

The synthetic estrogens and progestagens contained in the pills act in a way similar to that of the natural ovarian hormones—that is, by suppressing the production of stimulating hormones by the pituitary gland and thereby inhibiting the ovarian production of eggs.

Since the hormones in the pills are taken throughout the cycle, there is no possibility for the pituitary to escape their action and release ovarian stimulating factors. Without them, ovulation simply does not occur. Since the effect of these drugs is reversible—that is, when a woman stops taking them her body resumes its normal functions and its fertility—they can be used for contraceptive purposes.

I have heard that there is more than one kind of Pill. What is the difference?

Yes, two different types of oral contraceptive tablets are presently available. In the "combined" type, each tablet contains two kinds of hormonal drugs, an estrogen and a progestagen. In the "sequential" type the tablets are not all alike; they are taken in a special sequence of consecutive days, in which the estrogen is supplied throughout; the progestagen is added only toward the end of the cycle.

How are the pills taken?

They are supplied in packages containing a specific number of tablets, usually twenty (although there may be 21 or more to a monthly package), to be taken one a day, starting on the fifth day of the menstrual cycle, and continuing until the package is empty. When the last pill has been taken, the woman waits for a few days for her menstrual period to occur. The first day of menses is again counted as day one, and on day five she takes the first pill from a fresh package. If no menses appear, as can occasionally happen, she resumes taking the pills one week after having taken the last one from the previous package.

Doctors in the United States and elsewhere are trying to develop pills to be taken daily without interruption, since such continuous use will obviate the need for any counting at all.

What happens if a woman forgets to take a pill?

There is a chance that ovulation may occur if even one pill is missed, and she will run the risk of pregnancy. Therefore, if she misses one or more, while continuing to take the rest of her pills, she should be prepared to use some other contraceptive in addition, whenever intercourse occurs, until her next menstrual period.

Do these hormone drugs have any other effect on the body besides suppressing ovulation?

We have already mentioned that in some women menses may occasionally fail to appear. In most women, the amount of the menstrual flow decreases, and so do menstrual pain and premenstrual tension, while the cycles become more regular. On the other hand, a few women may find that slight bleeding or staining may occur unexpectedly while they are taking the pills; or they may experience some nausea at first. None of these symptoms is harmful, and they tend to disappear quite soon; but they should be reported to the physician who prescribed the pills. If they are at all persistent, he may change the prescription to one of a different formula which may be better tolerated by the individual, or advise another contraceptive method.

Can any woman take the Pill?

If her doctor approves, yes. Of course, no hormone drug should ever be taken without medical prescription. A physician prescribing an oral contraceptive will want to examine his patient at least twice a year. He will advise some other method of contraception if the woman is nursing a baby, or if she has any tendency or history of thrombophlebitis, inflammation of the veins, liver disease, diabetes, breast cancer or genital cancer, or if she is still adolescent. Also, if she has any fibroids in her uterus, the doctor may feel that is not advisable for her to take the pills, since the fibroids might get larger.

Is it safe to continue taking the Pill for more than two years?

Thousands of women are being studied to see if long-continued use of oral contraception is harmful in any way, and so far none of the suggested or suspected disadvantages has been confirmed, either in the women themselves or in their offspring. Normal fertility is not diminished, and the babies of mothers who have used the Pill are not affected by it.

Side Effects of the Pill

I have heard that the use of the Pill makes a woman fat. Is this true?

Many women taking the Pill will gain some weight. The action of the Pill resembles what goes on in the body of a woman in early pregnancy. One of the things that may occur in early pregnancy is water retention in the tissues, and this of course increases body weight. Although in some women there is a true gain in weight, this has been attributed to the sensation of well-being resulting from disappearance of the fear of pregnancy. However, the possibility of a true gain in body weight from the action of the Pill cannot be dismissed.

Some women actually lose weight while taking the Pill, although not so many as those who gain.

Water retention and weight changes, whatever the cause may be, usually occur during the first few months of taking the Pill.

You mentioned that bleeding may occur while a woman is taking the Pill. Is this different from menstruation?

Bleeding or staining while the Pill is being taken occurs in a good many women, especially during the early cycles—although not in all women, nor in all cycles. This bleeding in general is very light and usually lasts only a day or two, many times not even requiring the wearing of a sanitary napkin or a tampon; occasionally it may continue for several days. The reasons for such bleeding are unknown, but probably have something to do with the balance and action of the hormones produced by the woman's body in combination with those in the pills.

There is no agreement on how to overcome this problem. Some physicians may advise the woman to take two tablets rather than one a day, maybe one in the morning and one in the evening for as long as she bleeds. Others may advise her to take two tablets a day for the entire cycle. Still others may advise her to discontinue the tablets for a week and then start all over again. Most commonly, however, the doctor will advise his patient to continue taking the Pill regularly, as if nothing had happened, until all the tablets are finished, then to wait a week and start all over again.

There is no clear evidence as to which advice is best, but apparently a woman will have a better chance of recovering her regularity if she does not double the dose but continues taking the pills at the rate of one a day to the end of the cycle. Of course, since this bleeding is not related at all to the normal cyclic functions of the ovary when the woman did not take pills, this is not menstruation.

Are there any other side effects?

Yes; the most common is a sensation of nausea. This appears after a few days of taking the Pill and may last for a full cycle or even for several months. However, this may be overcome by taking the tablet after a meal, by not overloading the stomach, and perhaps by the use of unsweetened carbonated cold drinks. Vomiting is much rarer, but occasionally occurs during early experience with the Pill. Like nausea and most of the other symptoms that may accompany the taking of the Pill, this usually disappears in three to four months.

Some doctors may advise changing to another brand of pill to overcome some of the side effects, which may indeed disappear; but their disappearance may be due to the fact that the woman's body has become adjusted to the taking of these hormones rather than to the change of drugs.

Some women complain of bloating and swelling of the legs. This is also common in pregnancy, and may also disappear in a few months, although not necessarily so; in some women this problem may appear after many months of satisfactory use of the Pill.

A very common complaint by women using the Pill is breast tenderness. This is due to the reaction of the mammary-gland tissue to the stimulation of the hormones. Again, this closely resembles what occurs in early pregnancy, and breast tenderness and engorgement most commonly subside spontaneously after a few months.

Will the taking of the Pill affect the personality?

In our experience, most women get a sense of well-being they never experienced before; they will feel optimistic and euphoric. Others will not feel any different; a few will feel depressed. Such depression, again, may disappear spontaneously after a few months, although in some instances it may be necessary to discontinue the pills altogether.

Will sexual enjoyment be affected?

From time to time we hear that the Pill may decrease a woman's sexual enjoyment. In our experience, however, this problem has been infrequent. Most women will not be aware of any change in their sexual desire or in their ability to enjoy sex relations; many report that sexual enjoyment has begun only after they started taking the Pill. Of course, it is very difficult to evaluate the many psychological factors that may be involved in the enjoyment of the sexual act. For those whose sexual desires are diminished, one may argue that there may be some guilt feelings about suppressing the production of eggs, or even some fear of the effects of the drug. On the other hand, for those in whom sexual desire is increased or begun with the Pill, this may be due to relief from the fear of pregnancy.

In any case, the vast majority of women taking the Pill are satisfied with their sexual life.

The Pill and Cancer

Is there a connection between the pills and cancer? You say that the Pill is not advisable for women with cancer of the breast or of the genitals.

The reason for advising against the Pill for women who have had cancer is that sometimes cancer of the breast may be accelerated by the presence of estrogens; in some animal species tumors have appeared after the administration of high doses of these hormones. However, the hormone doses used in such animal studies have been much higher, in proportion to body size, than those used in the Pill for women; and tumors have appeared only in species that have a tendency to develop them spontaneously. All the studies in humans and in the most closely related animal species have failed to find any relationship between the prolonged taking of any of the hormones presently used in oral contraceptives and the development of cancer.

Uterine fibroids, which are often called uterine tumors, since for all doctors any mass is a tumor, may become larger when an oral contraceptive is used, but this is not always true. There is no evidence that the oral contraceptive may produce fibroids; but a previously undetected fibroid may become apparent, due mostly to the water retention produced by these drugs. This is another reason for the importance of the periodic medical checkup.

You may also occasionally hear that the oral pill may produce enlargement of the ovaries or the formation of cysts. This is not so, and goes against all basic and medical knowledge, since the ovaries are in a resting stage while the woman is on the Pill. Fibroids, which may also be present in the ovaries, of course, may grow under the action of the hormones in the Pill.

Women with premenstrual breast tenderness or pain in their breasts may experience a great deal of improvement with the use of the Pill. However, again, careful and periodic medical checkups are important.

I have heard that the Pill may have bad effects on the eyes. Is this true?

Some doctors have reported that some women have experienced changes in their vision. In all, these reports involve an almost negligible proportion of the over five million users in the United States alone, with almost as many in the rest of the world. We should always keep in mind, especially when we read newspaper headlines, that it is usually bad news which receives the most prominent coverage. Certainly the use of the Pill will not prevent the occurrence of diseases or problems which may affect the general population. The purpose of the Pill is to prevent conception, not to prevent disease.

Does use of the Pill make it harder for a woman to have a baby?

The Pill does not make any woman unable to have children. After stopping the Pill, the fertility of the woman returns almost immediately—certainly within three months—to what it was previously; and, although the data available are not too extensive, it appears that conception may occur even sooner after stopping the Pill than previously. Of course, we see women who stop the Pill and cannot conceive, but we should not forget that it is impossible to know what the previous fertility of these women was; many who use the Pill have never been pregnant before. We should remember also that fertility decreases with age. This is a toll that all humans pay, and for that reason it is always advisable for a couple who plan to have a family not to postpone too long the fulfillment of that desire.

Do you mean a woman may be more fertile after taking the Pill? Will she be more likely to have twins or triplets?

From time to time we read that a woman who formerly could not become pregnant did so after using the Pill for several months, not as a contraceptive but as a treatment for her fertility problem. Although this occurs, it is not so frequent as to allow us to state that the fertility of such a woman has improved because of the use of the Pill. This is referred to commonly as a "rebound effect" and is presently being studied.

As to the frequency of twins and other multiple births, we have not found at the Margaret Sanger Research Bureau that our clients who discontinue the Pill in order to conceive have experienced multiple pregnancies. It should always be remembered that multiple pregnancies occur more frequently nowadays, as we have mentioned previously; also, newspaper headlines make them more conspicuous. This question too is being carefully studied, and the information available so far does not support the contention that the increase in multiple births is related to the use of the Pill.

Is there any risk of abnormality in the children of a mother who has used the Pill?

Presently there is no evidence that the use of the Pill as a contraceptive will increase the danger of congenital malformation. Some years ago, it was reported that women who while they were pregnant had used similar drugs and even some of the same drugs as those contained in contraceptive pills, for the purpose of preventing a threatened miscarriage, delivered a number of female babies with some congenital abnormalities of the genital organs. These findings have not been encountered by other investigators and have been questioned by many. However, it should be remembered that these drugs are extremely potent, and that some of them, if given in high dosages very early in pregnancy, before the baby is completely formed (before the twelfth week of pregnancy), may produce this type of abnormality.

It is important also to remember that some of these hormones are actually used nowadays in very high doses to help women to continue with a pregnancy whose future was in danger, and many such women are able to carry to term without the baby showing any abnormality. We may say here that the factors related to drug-induced congenital abnormality include not only the drug given, but also the moment in the pregnancy, the dosage, and the length of administration.

Who Should Not Use the Pill

What circumstances would make it inadvisabe for a woman to take the Pill?

The prescription of the Pill to an adolescent girl—unless she has already had a baby—must be carefully weighed, since the hormones may stop normal growth of her body or may mask any possible abnormality in the establishment of her menstrual cycles. However, the physician must recognize and keep in mind also the dangers and consequences of an unwanted pregnancy at such an age which, aside from stopping the young mother's growth, may be quite tumultuous and the origin of many unfortunate social ills for her child.

Since we do not know as yet to what extent the hormones in the Pill may pass into the mother's milk or how they might then affect the child, it is advisable not to use them during the nursing period. Also, if the Pill is taken too early during the nursing period, it will diminish or stop the secretion of milk.

Before prescribing an oral contraceptive, the doctor will make a thorough examination of his patient's breasts, thyroid gland, legs and genital organs, and will make sure that in the past she has not suffered from thrombophlebitis or genital or breast cancer. If he finds any adverse condition, he may recommend some other method of contraception.

A history of liver or thyroid disease as well as the presence of diabetes, or the previous existence of this disease, does not preclude the use of the Pill; but the patient should be warned that her insulin requirements may increase, and that consequently she should be more closely supervised by her physician.

Contraception in the Future

Will you tell us what new contraceptive pills are likely to be used in the future?

Scientists are always on the lookout for better and simpler ways of achieving the same purpose. Presently a new sequential type of oral contraceptive is being studied; with this type, the pills are taken one a day without ever stopping. There is no waiting for menses, although they occur regularly; nor is there any counting to be done, which offers a great advantage. This method has proved to be highly acceptable and effective.

Another way of administering oral contraceptives that is presently being studied is to give the woman a very small dose of a very potent oral progestagen, which when administered daily, without stopping, will not inhibit ovulation; menses will occur more or less regularly. It is thought that it works by producing changes in the cervical mucus of the womb, although in some cases it has been proved that on frequent occasions it actually also stops ovulation. Although not as effective as the present oral contraceptives, this has proved an effective way of preventing pregnancy; and it may be more acceptable to groups now objecting to the use of the Pill, or even to women unable to use the presently available pills.

Other studies are being made of a pill containing estrogen alone, and also a new compound, the so-called "morning-after" pill, which, when taken by monkeys after mating, has proved to prevent pregnancy. These two approaches are presently being studied in humans on a very limited scale.

Compounds that can be stored by the body when taken orally will most likely be available also in the future, and these may provide us with a pill as effective as the present ones even when taken only once a month.

Of course, we can achieve the same purpose with some of the contraceptive drugs that now can be given by injection.

Contraceptive Injections

Please tell us about these contraceptive injections.

For several years we have had some hormones that, when given by injection, can be stored by the body and used over a long period of time. These drugs have been mostly used for the treatment of some cancer problems and for other therapeutic purposes. However, recently two similar preparations have been developed for the prevention of conception and are being extensively studied, here and abroad. One of these preparations contains, like the "combined" pill, an estrogen and a progestagen of long-term effect, which when injected once a month into a woman's body will suppress ovulation, though not menses. The other preparation contains only a progestagen, and when given by injection it will suppress ovulation, and usually also menses, for periods ranging from three to six or more months.

Neither of these preparations, however, is yet available for general use, although we have been using them both at the Sanger Bureau for almost two years and finding them highly acceptable and effective.

Are there any methods of preventing conception aside from the Pill, the intra-uterine devices, and the chemical and mechanical methods you mentioned?

Many different means are being explored; some of them, like the use of X rays on the testes, have been abandoned, since X rays not only arrest the capacity of the male glands to produce sperm—most of the time permanently—but also present some potential dangers. Besides, it is very difficult to adjust the dosage to assure complete arrest of sperm production while at the same time making sure that this arrest will be reversible. The skin of the scrotum also is very sensitive to X rays. These and some other undesirable effects have led to the abandonment of this method.

X rays also have been used for the suppression of ovulation; however, the ovaries are deep within a woman's body, they are much less sensitive to X rays than the male organs, and the dosages required are much higher. This produces some undesirable general body effects, and in many instances the ovaries will start producing eggs again. There is a possible danger that offspring of a woman who has had a large dose of X rays in order to suppress ovulation may have some congenital defects.

Heat applied locally to the testes has also been studied. As we have mentioned, there is a good reason why the human testes are outside the body, since normal body temperature is high enough to arrest the production of sperm. Repeated hot baths at temperatures around 100 degrees Fahrenheit and higher have been used in Japan with good results. Studies have also been made of the use of covered tight suspenders that, by insulating the scrotum and therefore diminishing the heat loss from it, keep the testes at the temperature of the body and thus gradually impair the production of sperm.

Is it true that conception might be controlled by vaccination?

For many years scientists have been working with this idea, and it is perfectly conceivable that in the future we may have vaccines that could be given to men or women in order to stop the production of sperm or otherwise make conception impossible. Of course, such a vaccine should not produce undesirable effects, and if reversible may be much more acceptable. Although great progress has been made in achieving temporary sterilization in male and female laboratory animals, the present methods are still unacceptable for human use.

The Ideal Contraceptive

What would you consider to be an ideal contraceptive?

The ideal contraceptive should first of all be harmless, without the likelihood of any injury to wife or husband or future offspring; it should be reliable and provide adequate protection; and it should be acceptable—that is, it should satisfy the individual needs of those who are to use it. This implies that the method should be simple, practical, inexpensive and aesthetically satisfying. Although the Pill and the intra-uterine devices very closely approach all these requirements, the ideal contraceptive still remains to be developed.

Contraception is no longer a controversial subject; religious and political leaders recognize not only the dangers of overpopulation of the world, but, just as important, the danger of overpopulation in individual families, which is much more acute and promptly acknowledged. Family limitation has been practiced for many years despite the fact that many people didn't talk about it. Infanticide, abortion, abandonment of children have gone on for longer than recorded history. Fortunately now it is generally recognized that a pregnancy should be a wanted pregnancy, and that couples should decide for themselves the number of offspring they want to have; in fact, we are starting to hear that the timing of pregnancy is a woman's privilege, and that nobody but she should decide when she should bear a child. This recognition of willed or voluntary parenthood as a woman's right and the acknowledgment of contraception and its individual and social importance led to a salutary upsurge of research in reproductive physiology at all levels. Out of all this work, we can expect a better knowledge of ourselves and of the processes leading to conception and how to control them.

Sterilization

Will you tell us about sterilization?

Sterilization is not a method of contraception, of course. It makes a man or a woman permanently incapable of reproduction. As we mentioned previously, this can be achieved by the use of X ray in either the male or the female, but this is not a desirable method. The only practical and approved methods in use at the present time are the surgical ones. The surgical procedure consists in producing an artificial obstruction to the passage of the sperm cells in the case of the male, or of the egg cells in the case of the female.

Sterilization of the Male (Vasectomy)

In the male it is the vas deferens, the tube that carries the sperm from the testes and epididymus to the penis, which is blocked for this purpose. You will recall that in order to reach the outside the sperm have to pass through the seminal duct, or vas, which runs from the testes through the groin and then backward into the urinary channel. If these ducts are cut or tied, the sperm will be unable to pass through. This operation is called vasectomy. As the bulk of the seminal fluid comes from the seminal vesicles and the prostate, the ejaculations will continue in a fairly normal manner and quantity, but the seminal fluid will not contain any sperm, and the individual will be rendered sterile. The operation is comparatively simple, because in the scrotum and the groin the vas lies close to the surface. It can be performed under a local anesthetic as an office procedure, and it requires virtually no rest.

I thought that sterilization involved the removal of the sex glands, and that a sterilized individual would lose all sexual feelings.

No, sterilization does not involve the removal of the testes or of the ovaries; the sex glands are not affected at all. The operation merely stops the migration of the egg or the sperm and renders the individual incapable of reproduction, but it does not diminish the sexual desire or the capacity to have a normal sex life, nor does it produce any adverse physical or psychic changes.

Sterilization of the Female

What operation is performed on a woman to make her sterile?

In the woman the Fallopian tubes are usually cut and tied off, after which the eggs from the ovaries cannot reach the uterus, nor can the sperm gain access to the egg. An operation of this kind requires an abdominal incision and hospitalization for a few days, and it is therefore a more involved undertaking than sterilization of the man.

A simplified method of blocking the tubes which does not require an abdominal incision has also been used. A special instrument is introduced through the vagina or through a small opening near the umbilicus into the abdomen, and both Fallopian tubes are closed with a metal clip or by coagulating the tissues with an electric current.

But suppose the man or woman desires children later on—is it possible to reopen the passages?

Operations to reunite the cut ends of the seminal ducts or the Fallopian tubes at a later date have been successful in few instances. In the main, however, when the ducts or tubes are cut the individual must be considered permanently sterile. Therefore it is best to resort to sterilization only where permanent sterility is indicated or desired.

In recent years studies have been made of a surgical procedure by which small clips are placed on the Fallopian tubes. Through a small puncture made in the posterior wall of the vagina, a thin instrument called a culdoscope is introduced into the abdominal cavity; through it the gynecologist is able to see the tubes and place the clips on them. It is hoped, though not yet proved that, since they produce only minimal lesions, the clips may be removed and the tubes' normal function restored, if desired.

More recently, scientists working with experimental animals in the laboratory have been using the injection of a very small amount of a synthetic rubber into the vas deferens of the male, with the idea that this substance, which is very well tolerated by the tissues, may later be surgically removed and fertility restored.

Under what circumstances is sterilization advisable, Doctor?

Sterilization may be indicated on medical, eugenic or social grounds. When a pregnancy is likely to endanger the life of a woman, and permanent protection against conception is necessary, sterilization may be the method of choice. It may, in fact, be the best procedure to follow from a medical viewpoint.

Then there is the need for the permanent control of procreation among those afflicted with hereditary defects. There is general agreement among scientists that individuals suffering from hereditary physical and mental disabilities should avoid reproduction, first because of the possibility of the transmission of the defect, and secondly because mentally handicapped parents are not likely to give their children the care needed for their physical and emotional development. When such individuals are incapable of employing the available contraceptive methods, operative sterilization affords a humane, practicable and effective measure.

In addition to the strictly medical and eugenic indications, social conditions may at times also constitute a valid reason for sterilization. When a couple have had all the children they can rear adequately and usefully, when they have had all the children they would wish, and further childbearing is definitely no longer contemplated, the husband or the wife may seek to be sterilized. Sterilization eliminates the need for the use of contraceptive measures and provides protection from conception for the remaining years of their reproductive life.

Sterilizations in the United States

Aren't there some states that have enacted laws for the sterilization of individuals afflicted with hereditary diseases?

The United States was the first country in the world to enact a eugenic sterilization law, and at present approximately half of the states have valid sterilization statutes of one kind or another. These statutes generally provide for the compulsory sterilization of individuals who are insane or feeble-minded and who have been committed to state institutions. The first sterilization statute was adopted in 1907 by the state of Indiana. Two years later, in 1909, California,

Connecticut and Washington adopted somewhat similar legislation, and since then a large number of other states have passed eugenic sterilization laws. Several of these laws, however, were later declared to be invalid by the courts.

Are many compulsory eugenic sterilizations being performed in this country at present?

About twenty years ago, approximately two thousand such sterilizations were performed annually in the United States, and a little over fifty thousand persons, more than half of them women, had been officially sterilized. However, there has been a steady decline in the number of such operations. A survey in 1963 indicated that fewer than five hundred such operations were performed in the United States during that year. In most states an order for sterilization can be appealed for review to a state eugenics board and then, if necessary, to a court of law.

Do the sterilization laws apply only to people who are mentally defective or insane?

Well, the grounds for legal sterilization differ in various states. In most of them the laws are strictly eugenic in character and are intended only to prevent the transmission of hereditary diseases, but in a few states other grounds are also recognized. In several, for example, "habitual criminality" is also mentioned in the statutes as a ground for sterilization, making the law not only eugenic but also punitive in character.

But should such a step be forced upon anybody as a punishment?

When intended as a punishment for criminal acts, sterilization is clearly a dangerous social policy. In several states such laws have been declared by the courts to be unconstitutional, on the basis that sterilization is an "unusual and cruel" punishment for a criminal offense.

An interesting example of the dangers of such a law occurred in Oklahoma. In 1935 the state of Oklahoma passed a eugenic sterilization law which, among other things, provided for the compulsory sterilization of any person adjudged to be a "habitual criminal." The term "habitual criminal" was defined to mean a person convicted three or more times of the commission of crimes involving moral turpitude. In 1941 a man with three convictions, one of them for chicken stealing, which is regarded in Oklahoma as a crime involving moral turpitude, was ordered to be sterilized. The convicted man appealed the order, and the case finally came before the United States Supreme Court, which ruled unanimously that the Oklahoma statute was unconstitutional. In writing the opinion, Justice Douglas pointed out that this legislation involved one of the basic civil rights of man, and that the power to sterilize "may have subtle, far-reaching and devastating effects." The Supreme Court apparently did not object to eugenic sterilization as such, but rather to its potential abuses. Such abuses are apt to arise when a law fails to limit its application only to conditions which, on the basis of modern scientific knowledge, are known to be hereditary, or when it fails to safeguard the rights of the individual to judicial appeal.

But even in cases of sterilization for eugenic reasons, is it necessary that the laws be compulsory?

No, I feel that even when the laws are strictly eugenic in character, they should be voluntary rather than compulsory in nature. The resort to wide-scale enforced sterilization, as was practiced, for example, in Germany during the Nazi regime, is, of course, an arbitrary and unwarranted assumption of power by the state. In the United States, it is true, compulsion, as I mentioned before, is rarely employed in practice, and usually the written consent either of the patient or of the nearest relative or guardian is obtained. Nevertheless, the laws should be so worded that the rights of the individual are adequately protected.

In democratic countries coercive measures are contrary to public sentiment. Greater progress can certainly be made at present by voluntary measures rather than compulsory statutes. Under wise and humane control sterilization can serve a useful purpose.

What about voluntary sterilization?

Voluntary sterilization is legal in all fifty states, although only five states make mention of such a procedure in their laws. In the other states no mention is made of it in the laws, hence there is no prohibition. Utah and Connecticut permit voluntary sterilization, but restrict it to reasons of medical necessity. Virginia, North Carolina and Georgia have affirmative laws which permit voluntary sterilization and spell out legal and medical procedures that must be followed. At the present time about two million Americans have been voluntarily sterilized and over 100,000 obtain such operations annually.

Why should people wish to be sterilized?

As I mentioned, when childbearing may endanger the life or health of the woman, sterilization may be preferred to the use of contraceptive measures because it provides greater certainty of protection. A woman who, for instance, has had three or more Caesarean sections may well wish to have her tubes tied in order to avoid subjecting herself to the dangers of further operations. Sometimes it is the husband who seeks the sterilization under these circumstances. Then again, a person suffering from a hereditary disease may be anxious to avoid any possibility of transmitting the disease to a future generation. He might consider himself fit for marriage and yet unfit for reproduction.

There are also some people who want to be sterilized because they feel that they already have a sufficiently large family and do not want to rely upon or cannot employ the usual contraceptive methods. Havelock Ellis advocated the use of sterilization for three types of cases: where there are already a sufficient number of children in the family, where the wife's failing health renders it undesirable to have more children, or where it is undesirable ever to have any children at all, a classification which includes medical and eugenic as well as social indications.

What is your opinion of such voluntary sterilization, Doctor?

A sterilization should be resorted to only when procreation must be permanently avoided. When there are valid medical or eugenic reasons for such a procedure, a man or woman should have the privilege of having this operation performed. It is not at all advisable, however, in my opinion, for anyone to seek a sterilization merely because this provides a less troublesome or more certain means for the prevention of conception. Sterilization should still be considered an irreversible step, and there are so many unpredictable possibilities in life that one should exercise great caution and deliberation before submitting to such an operation. Merely for family-planning purposes, the use of a medically chosen contraceptive provides ample protection.

I understand there are various kinds of drugs that are taken to stop a pregnancy. Are they really effective?

I know of no drugs available at present which can be used for the purpose of interrupting a pregnancy. Drugs are frequently taken or prescribed for a delayed menstrual period, but a delay does not necessarily denote a pregnancy. Any number of physical or psychic conditions, such as exposure to sudden changes of temperature, bodily ailments, debility, an unbalanced diet, disturbances of the glandular functions, emotional strain and worry, may cause a delay of the menstrual flow for days or even weeks. In a group of one thousand women who were examined at the Margaret Sanger Research Bureau because of menstrual delays ranging from a few days to weeks, we found that over sixty-five per cent of them were not pregnant at all, and eventually they had normal periods. Hormones are prescribed in such cases to correct the underlying condition and to restore the menstrual rhythm, but when the cessation of the menstruation is due to a conception, medication has no effect. The usual pills or liquids, containing ergot or various other chemical and vegetable compounds, which are sold for the purpose of inducing an abortion are of no value if the woman is really pregnant and a normal embryo has already implanted itself in the uterus.

Abortions

How is a pregnancy interrupted?

When we discuss the problems of fertility, we will talk about "spontaneous" abortions, or involuntary terminations of pregnancy. Now we are talking about the deliberate interruption of a pregnancy, usually in its early stages. This type of abortion is generally a surgical operation which involves the removal of the embryo from the uterus. The lower end of the uterus is first dilated, and then the fertilized ovum with its surrounding tissues is removed by a surgical instrument known as a curette. The operation itself is called a curettage, and it is a surgical procedure which requires an anesthetic. Recently a new surgical procedure for aborting unwanted pregnancies has been incorporated into some hospitals here and abroad. It consists of utilizing a special hollow cannula in the pregnant uterus during the first few weeks of pregnancy. By applying high vacuum, the products of conception are removed in a very short time and apparently with many fewer problems for the woman.

In the later stages of pregnancy a therapeutic abortion may be performed by the injection of certain solutions directly through the abdomen and the uterus into the sac of fluid which surrounds the fetus. This leads to the interruption of the pregnancy, and the fetus is spontaneously aborted shortly after. The method is being studied in this country, although in a very restricted and cautious way.

Legal and Illegal Abortions

When are induced abortions legal?

Legal, or "therapeutic," abortions may be performed in some countries in the following situations: (1) where the pregnancy threatens the life of the mother; (2) in cases of rape, incest, etc.; (3) where there is danger of congenital malformation in the infant because of disease or harmful drugs in the mother; or (4) where the birth of a child would constitute a socioeconomic threat to the mother. In this country, a few states have enacted laws legalizing abortions in the first three situations, but none has accepted the fourth.

Does this mean that not many abortions are performed in this country?

Far from it. Abortion as a way of family limitation has always been practiced quite widely. Because most of the induced abortions performed in this country are illegal, the exact figures cannot be determined, but it is estimated that in the United States between two hundred thousand and one and a half million unwanted pregnancies are terminated in this way every year.

Contrary to what most people believe, most of the illegal abortions are not performed on unmarried women. Mothers who already have as many children as they can care for are all too frequently the victims of this social blight when they find themselves pregnant again. The social problem of abortion is fortunately being aired vigorously nowadays, and it is to be hoped that in the not too distant future most of the states of the Union will pass sensible laws permitting and regulating the practice of legal abortion.

One of the reasons for the present interest in the subject is the recognition that voluntary terminations of pregnancy have been possible without risk for those who can afford them. Women with sufficient means are able to secure the help of an understanding surgeon or physician who can perform the operation under hospital conditions, when not in a hospital, while the economically deprived groups having the same problems, desires and motivation have to expose themselves to amateurish hands. More than eight out of every ten maternal deaths among the economically deprived are due to consequences of voluntary termination of pregnancy.

Are abortions dangerous or injurious?

In this country alone an estimated two thousand women die annually, and a very much larger number become chronically ill, as the result of abortions. Many women become sterile following such operations. This high death and sickness rate is due in part to the fact that most of the abortions are carried out secretly, often under very unsanitary conditions and by untrained and incompetent individuals. Some are even induced by the pregnant women themselves, an especially dangerous procedure. Under such circumstances injuries and infections are very apt to occur. When the operation is performed by a trained surgeon under strictly aseptic conditions the dangers are very much reduced. As a matter of fact, it is less dangerous in regard to the life of the mother than pregnancy itself. Nevertheless, the interruption of a pregnancy is never a slight matter and may be accompanied by considerable physical and psychic shock to the woman.

The Status of Abortion in the Soviet Union and Japan

Are there any countries where it is legal to have an abortion even if there are no special medical indications?

In Russia in 1920, not long after the Soviet regime came into power, abortions were legalized. This step was taken, it was claimed then, primarily as a public-health measure—to safeguard the health of women who, because of the very difficult social and economic conditions of the time, were already resorting in large numbers to the interruption of pregnancies. For the protection of the health of the women, the Soviet authorities decided to bring this underground practice into the open so that it could be adequately supervised and controlled. Special government hospitals were set aside where a woman in need of an abortion could have the operation performed by trained physicians and under strictly sanitary conditions. The patient was required to remain in the hospital for three days following the operation. However, a pregnancy was not to be interrupted if it had advanced beyond the third month, nor when a woman was pregnant for the first time, unless there were urgent social indications or serious danger to her health.

This law did serve to decrease to a considerable degree the number of deaths and other complications following abortions. Nevertheless, it became evident after a time that even under the best hospital conditions abortions were not always without danger or subsequent harm to the health of the women, and that the large-scale resort to the interruption of pregnancies led to many physical disabilities. As a result, a widespread educational campaign was instituted by the public-health authorities to acquaint the people with the nature and the dangers of abortion and with the advisability of preventing conceptions rather than resorting to the interruption of pregnancy. In 1936 the Soviet government rescinded the legalization of abortion, partly for medical reasons, because of the resulting complications, and partly, no doubt, because of a growing emphasis on a larger population, owing to the changing social and political conditions at the time. However, after World War II the government reverted to its original policy. In general, abortions are permitted throughout Eastern Europe with the exception of East Germany and Rumania.

In Japan, abortions on economic grounds were legalized in 1948. As a result, the number of such operations in that country increased from 246,000 in 1949 to 1,128,000 in 1958, but this has now declined to approximately one million annually. The public-health authorities of Japan realize the seriousness of the situation and are trying to take active measures to expand their birth-control activities.

Abortion Law in Sweden

What about the Scandinavian countries?

The Scandinavian countries are attempting to solve the abortion problem through a progressive social and medical approach. In Sweden, for example, a number of official consultation bureaus have been established for women seeking abortions. Any woman who desires to have her pregnancy interrupted may apply to one of these bureaus for consultation and assistance. There her individual situation is considered, and an attempt is made to help her adjust her personal and family problems to enable her to continue with her pregnancy. If needed, economic assistance for immediate relief is provided. At the same time she is also informed about the risks involved in abortion, and every effort is made to deter her from interfering with the pregnancy. If she persists in her determination, she is referred to a special medical board for a final decision. Therapeutic indications for interrupting a pregnancy have been extended in Sweden to include not only strictly medical but also medicosocial grounds. Abortions are permitted in cases where, because of social conditions and other circumstances, the health of a woman might be seriously harmed by the birth and care of an additional child. The board considers the various factors in each case, and it has the power to sanction or refuse a legal abortion on the basis of these broader indications.

Social and Medical Aspects of Abortion

Do you think that it will be possible to stop the resort to abortions altogether?

The question of abortions is not purely a medical one; it is intimately bound up with our social, moral, ethical and religious views, and the problem cannot be solved without a considerable social and ethical reorientation. It seems obvious, however, that our present restrictive measures have failed in their purpose and that other means will have to be adopted. First, it seems to me that adequate social, economic and medical aid ought to be provided for potential parents so that all pregnancies will be wanted and planned. A wanted pregnancy is never voluntarily interrupted.

Second, we might extend the scope of the medicolegal indications for abortion, somewhat along the lines adopted in countries with more progressive legislation. At the present time it is legally permissible to interrupt a pregnancy only if it places the life of the mother in danger. There are, however, many medical, eugenic and even social conditions which, though they do not exactly endanger the life of the woman, definitely contraindicate a pregnancy on physical or psychological grounds, and such conditions might well be considered as therapeutic indications for abortions. An extension of the indications for pregnancy interruptions, under adequate social and medical control, would bring this practice into greater harmony with present-day public opinion and mores.

A measure for the control of abortion which I believe to be of paramount importance would be the wide dissemination of information about contraception. If every woman were supplied with adequate and reliable contraceptive knowledge, the incidence of abortion would be greatly decreased. The prevention of abortions can be most effectively achieved by the prevention of unwanted conceptions.

Bibliography

Bromley, Dorothy D., *Catholics and Birth Control*. Devin, 1965.

Burgess, Ernest W., and Fishbein, Morris, M.D., eds., *Successful Marriage*, rev. ed. Doubleday, 1955.

Calderone, Mary S., M.D., ed., *Manual of Contraceptive Practice*. Williams and Wilkins, 1964.

Day, Richard L., M.D., *Fertility Control: A Social Need—A Medical Responsibility*. Planned Parenthood/World Population, 1966.

Dickinson, Robert L., M.D., *Techniques of Conception Control*, 3rd ed. Williams and Wilkins, 1950. Also in paperback.

Fletcher, Joseph, *Morals and Medicine*. Beacon Press paperback, 1960.

Guttmacher, Alan F., M.D., *The Case for Legalized Abortion Now.* Diablo Press, 1967.

——, *The Consumers Union Report on Family Planning,* 2nd ed. Consumers Union of the U.S., 1966.

——, with Winfield Best and Frederick S. Jaffe, *The Complete Book of Birth Control,* Ballantine, 1961.

Himes, Norman E., *A Medical History of Contraception.* Gamut (Taplinger), 1964.

——, and Stone, Abraham, M.D., *Planned Parenthood—A Practical Guide to Birth Control Methods.* Collier paperback, 1964.

Holden, Raymond T., M.D., Chairman, The Committee on Human Reproduction of the American Medical Association, "The Control of Fertility," *Journal of the American Medical Association,* Vol. 194, pp. 462–470 (Oct. 25, 1965).

Lader, Lawrence, *Abortion.* Bobbs-Merrill, 1966.

Rock, John, M.D., *The Time Has Come.* Knopf, 1963.

Smith, David T., ed., *Abortion and the Law.* Press of Western Reserve University, 1967.

Suenens, Leon J., *Love and Control.* Newman, 1961.

Thomas, John L., S.J., *Marriage and Rhythm.* Newman, 1957.

Williams, Glanville, *The Sanctity of Life and the Criminal Law.* Knopf, 1957.

CHAPTER VI

FERTILITY AND INFERTILITY

Today, I should like to discuss with you a little more fully several other aspects of human fertility and infertility which are of practical importance in marriage.

Fertility

I am not quite certain, Doctor, what you mean by the term "fertility."

By "fertility" I mean the ability to beget offspring. Not all couples, obviously, possess this capacity to the same degree. Some are very fruitful, with numerous progeny; others have only a few children; and some remain childless altogether.

Factors Influencing Fertility

Aren't the differences in the number of children in a family usually due to the use of birth-control measures?

Not necessarily. I am referring to variations in the fertility of couples even when no contraceptive measures are used. There are many factors, both hereditary and environmental, which affect the fertility of an individual. Darwin pointed out long ago that domestic animals breed faster than wild animals of the same species, and he ascribed this to the effects of a more ample and regular food supply. On the other hand, wild animals in captivity frequently do not breed at all. It has also been shown that in animals, at least, the absence from the diet of certain vitamins or other essential factors may cause a diminution or complete loss of fertility. In humans, too, diet and general bodily health appear to have a very definite effect upon reproductive capacity. Then, of course, age, especially of the woman, is a significant factor in fertility, and it influences to a very marked degree her capacity to beget offspring.

Adolescent Sterility

How long does a woman's childbearing period last?

The reproductive span of a woman extends from puberty to the menopause—in general, from age fifteen to age forty-five. It has generally been assumed that a girl becomes fertile as soon as she begins to menstruate. However, the onset of menses does not necessarily imply capacity for reproduction. The ripening of the egg cells may not begin until some time after the menses have been established. This interval between the first appearance of the menstrual flow and the beginning of the capacity to conceive and reproduce has been called the period of "adolescent sterility," and it may vary from several months to one or two years. During this period conception is not impossible, but it is not likely to occur.

Normally, a girl becomes capable of bearing a child some time between the ages of twelve and fifteen. Rare instances have been recorded of pregnancies in much younger girls—girls of ten, nine and even six. In 1939 an Indian girl from Peru was reported to have been delivered of a normal child by Caesarean section at the age of five and a half years. Such cases, however, are very unusual.

A woman's fertility comes to an end when her menses cease and when she reaches her "change of life," or the menopause. As the age at which this occurs is variable, the duration of a woman's fertility varies correspondingly. Usually reproductive capacity ceases in the mid-forties, although exceptional cases of childbirth in the late fifties and even sixties have been reported now and then.

Age and Female Fertility

To what extent does the age of a woman affect her chances of pregnancy? Is it more difficult for her to conceive later in life?

The 1960 census reported that about eighty-two percent of American children are born to women between the ages of twenty and thirty-nine, and only eighteen per cent to mothers under twenty or over thirty-nine. It is generally accepted that the fertility of a woman starting at puberty rises gradually to its height in the twenties and then diminishes, at first slowly and then more rapidly. With the onset of the menopause, in the forties, fertility decreases at a faster rate, and the chances of a conception are correspondingly reduced.

Is there any basis for the belief that some women become more fertile during the "change of life"?

Perhaps you recall the story of Sarah, who, according to the Bible, conceived for the first time at the full age of ninety, long after "it had ceased to be with her after the manner of women." This story might be quite plausible if the Biblical year was, as some maintain, half the length of our own, for occasionally a pregnancy does occur toward the end of the menopause.

The menopause comes on rather gradually, and it takes several years before the process is completed. The menses do not cease at once, but become more and more irregular, with a gradual increase in the interval between successive periods. While a pregnancy is not very likely to occur during these years of "change," it is not impossible. Hence it is a time of great anxiety for many women, for with the menstrual irregularities they are often puzzled to know whether the cessation of the menses is the result of menopausal changes or of a possible impregnation. To avoid the recurring uncertainties of this period, it is advisable to continue the use of contraceptive measures until a year has passed without a menstrual flow.

Age and Male Fertility

Is the fertility of a man also influenced by his age?

A boy, too, first becomes fertile when he reaches puberty, which usually occurs between the ages of fifteen and eighteen. It is at this time that the sperm cells begin to be formed in the testes, and that he becomes capable of a seminal emission which can cause impregnation. His fertility, however, lasts much later in life than that of the woman. Cases of men who become fathers at sixty and even seventy are not infrequent. A case of a man who was fertile at ninety-seven has been reported in the medical literature. It is likely, however, that the fertility of men also lessens as they pass beyond their middle age in life.

Sterility or Infertility

You spoke before about some couples having no children. Are there many childless marriages?

The census report of 1960 showed that fourteen per cent of all married women in the United States never bear any children. Most of this childlessness is probably involuntary, for not many couples choose to remain without children throughout their married life. Exact statistics on the incidence of sterility are, however, difficult to obtain, for sterility may be primary, when no children at all are born to a couple, or it may be secondary—that is, when no children come after one or more have already been born. In such cases the marriage would no longer be reported as childless in the census records.

As a matter of fact, we now prefer to use the term "infertility" rather than "sterility" in cases of childlessness. "Sterility" implies a more or less permanent inability to beget offspring, but many barren couples can be rendered fertile by means of modern medical measures.

When is a marriage regarded as infertile? I mean, how long a period must elapse without a pregnancy before a marriage is considered barren?

While a conception may follow a single sexual contact, the first pregnancy, even when no preventive measures are used, may not occur for several months after regular sexual relations have been established, and sometimes not for several years. One cannot, therefore, tell with certainty when a marriage is to be considered infertile. However, it is not advisable to wait longer than a year before seeking medical aid. If a woman is over thirty, it is not advisable to wait more than half a year. Medical help should also be sought promptly when there is menstrual irregularity or any suspicion that previous or existing disease may have altered the reproductive ability of either spouse.

The Causes of Infertility

What is usually the cause of childlessness, Doctor?

Let us briefly review the essential steps in reproduction. For a fruitful conception to occur it is necessary, first, that an adequate supply of healthy sperm be deposited in the genital tract of the female at or near the opening of the cervix; second, that the passages through the cervical canal, the uterus and the Fallopian tubes be free for the sperm to ascend; and, third, that a healthy ovum be present in the tube where the union of the sperm and ovum occurs. In addition, the lining of the uterus must be sufficiently well-developed to offer a suitable place for the implantation and development of the fertilized ovum. Disturbances in any of these essential conditions, on the part of either the man or the woman, may lead to impairment of fertility.

Then in a case of childlessness either the husband or the wife may be at fault?

Yes, that is quite true. As a matter of fact, one of the most significant recent advances in the study of fertility has been the realization that the fruitfulness of a marriage depends upon the degree of fertility of both mates, and that the responsibility for childlessness must be shared by both husband and wife. Formerly, it was the woman who was nearly always considered responsible for a sterile mating, and even today we are most apt to regard her as being at fault when a union proves to be childless. Barrenness has always been looked upon not only as an unfortunate circumstance, but also as a cause for reproach to the woman. In some countries sterility is a cause for divorce, and the childless woman is regarded with contempt and scorn. It is only within comparatively recent years that the male factor in the causation of sterile marriages has come to be appreciated more fully. Today we find that in a high percentage of childless unions, variously estimated as from thirty to fifty per cent, it is the husband who is deficient in fertility. As a matter of fact, the present viewpoint is that the fruitfulness of any particular marriage does not depend solely upon the condition of either the husband or the wife, but rather upon the degrees of fertility of both of them.

Is it possible that a man and a woman may not be able to have children with each other and yet beget offspring with other mates?

Yes, that may happen. Instances of this kind are due in the main to the fact that fertility is not an absolute quality, and that a man or a woman need not necessarily be either completely fertile or completely sterile. There are many varying degrees of reproductive capacity. If both mates happen to have a low fertility, they may be unable to have children with each other, yet if each one should remarry a mate with a high grade of fertility, the subsequent unions may prove to be normally fruitful.

Infertility of the Male

What are the causes of a lack of fertility in the husband?

The function of the male in reproduction is to deposit active and healthy sperm at the entrance to the uterus. If the husband is unable to deposit his seminal fluid into the genital tract of the wife, or if his sperm are defective in quantity or quality, his wife will not conceive.

Inability to carry the semen into the vagina may be due either to some congenital malformation of the male organ or to a lack of adequate sexual potency. If the husband's erection is not firm enough to effect penetration, or if he ejaculates before entry has been accomplished, conception is not likely to occur.

Such cases, however, are comparatively infrequent. Usually male infertility is due to an inadequacy of the seminal fluid. You will recall that the sperm are formed in the testes and from there they pass through a rather complex series of ducts in the epididymis and the vas deferens until they are ejaculated in the semen. Each seminal emission consists on an average of about a teaspoonful, or four cubic centimeters, of fluid, which is made up largely of secretions from the prostate and the seminal vesicles. Within this fluid are also the sperm, from fifty to one hundred million per cubic centimeter, or a total of some two to four hundred million in a single emission. Normal and healthy sperm have a characteristic form and can remain alive for some twenty-four to seventy-two hours. A decrease in the number of sperm to much below forty million per cubic centimeter, a diminution in the degree or duration of their vitality, or the presence of many abnormal forms would be indicative of a diminished fertility.

Azoospermia

Are there special tests or studying the quality of the seminal fluid?

Yes, methods have been developed for an accurate determination of the quantity and quality of the sperm in the seminal fluid. It is now possible to count the number of sperm in an ejaculation, to study the degree of their vitality, and to examine their form and structure. As a matter of fact, the movements and the shapes of the sperm as seen through the microscope have even been photographed as an aid in semen analysis.

In some cases the seminal fluid contains no sperm at all, a condition known as azoospermia. This may result either from a failure of the testes to produce any sperm or from obstructions in the seminal ducts which prevent the sperm cells from passing through.

What may cause a failure of sperm production?

Lack of sperm formation may be caused by a variety of conditions. Congenital abnormalities such as undescended testes, disturbances of the pituitary or thyroid glands which in turn affect the testes, dietary deficiencies, exposure of the testes to X rays, infections of the genital organs or even general systemic diseases—any of these may seriously affect sperm production.

Among the general infectious diseases, mumps is of special importance. If it occurs during or after puberty, it is sometimes complicated by an inflammation of one or both testes, which may later lead to an atrophy of these glands and to a loss of their sperm-forming function.

Then again, as I mentioned, the sperm may be formed normally, but they may be blocked somewhere along the route. Such blockages may be caused by a congenital malformation, by an injury, or by a gonorrheal or other infection of the ducts leading from the testes.

If one testicle is injured and does not function, how does it affect the man's fertility?

One testis, if it is in normal condition, is quite sufficient to produce all the sperm required for impregnation. Many men have fathered children even though one of their testes was undescended, atrophied, or blocked.

Testicular Biopsy

In cases where there are no sperm in the semen, is there any way of telling whether it is due to a lack of sperm production or to some obstruction?

To find out whether the absence of sperm is the result of a failure of sperm formation or the result of an obstruction, a minor operation, known as a testicular biopsy, can be performed. A minute portion of testicular tissue is removed for a microscopic examination which shows whether the testes are functioning normally or not. If they are not producing any sperm at all, the chances of a cure are very remote. For the present, at least, we have no means of restoring the sperm-forming function of the testes, although active research is being continued in this field. If the sperm production is partially impaired, various medical treatments may be attempted. If, however, the examination of the tissue shows that the testes are functioning normally, then the absence of sperm from the seminal fluid is, in all probability, due to a blockage somewhere along their route. This condition can be corrected in some instances by a surgical procedure which reopens the duct for the passage of the cells.

Sperm Deficiencies

When a man is sterile, then, Doctor, is it usually due to an absence of sperm cells?

No, cases of complete azoospermia account for only a small percentage of male sterility. Out of a hundred childless couples, some eight or ten of the husbands may show azoospermia. In most instances, impaired fertility of the husband is due not to a complete absence of sperm, but to a deficiency either in their number, their vitality or their quality. Such deficiencies may result from many causes—from glandular disturbances, nutritional disorders, vitamin deficiencies, general or local infections—in fact, from any condition that depresses the physiological functioning of the body. The process of sperm production is a very complex and delicate function and is readily affected by bodily disorders. It appears to rise or fall with the general level of health.

Sometimes men in apparently excellent health have deficient seminal fluids, and even a thorough investigation fails to show the cause. Many of the factors which lead to a decrease or loss of sperm production and to diminution of fertility are still unknown.

If the semen is deficient in either the number or the quality of the sperm, can anything be done to improve it?

That would depend upon the cause. If the deficiency is due to poor nutrition, glandular disturbances or the presence of some local or general infection, then appropriate treatment with vitamins, hormones and other special medications may be of great value. When, however, the testicular function has been seriously damaged, little can be done at present. In general, our knowledge of the factors which are responsible for semen deficiencies is still inadequate, and the treatment of such conditions is not very satisfactory. At times, however, the semen may improve markedly as a result of general changes in the life pattern of the individual, without any special treatment at all.

Infertility of the Female

When the husband is fertile, Doctor, and the childlessness is due to the wife, what are the causes likely to be?

Among the chief factors in female sterility are failure of ovulation, obstructions in the genital tract, especially in the cervix or the Fallopian tubes, and disturbances in the development of the uterus and its lining which interfere with the implantation and growth of the fertilized ovum.

Can the quality of the egg cells be studied the way that of the sperm can?

No, we have no definite means of ascertaining the quality or vitality of a woman's egg cells as we do in the case of the sperm. The ova are, of course, not accessible to direct examination, and their condition has to be determined indirectly from a general study of the woman and of her reproductive system.

Are there some women who do not produce any egg cells at all, just as some men produce no sperm?

Yes, there are. You will recall that normally one ovum ripens during each month. Occasionally, however, the egg cell may fail to mature at all, or, if it does mature, it may not be released from the ovary.

Determining the Time of Ovulation

Is it possible to tell, then, whether a woman produces egg cells or not?

Several methods are now available for determining the occurrence and the time of ovulation. During our discussion of the safe period, we spoke of the value of the daily temperature record in telling when a woman ovulates. A chart of the daily waking temperature over a period of several months provides a fairly simple and quite accurate method for telling whether and approximately when a woman ovulates. This record can be used by childless couples to establish the days of maximum fertility. Daily temperature records are now used quite extensively in the study of infertility, and they have proven to be of much aid both in diagnosis and in treatment.

The time of ovulation can also be told by the study of the secretion that comes from the cervix, the so-called "cervical mucus." Around the time that the ovum is being released, this secretion becomes more profuse and thinner in consistency, and if it is allowed to dry and is examined under the microscope it shows some crystals shaped like palm or fern leaves; in a normal woman, this indicates that ovulation is about to take place.

The study of vaginal cells by the vaginal-smear method is another valuable aid in determining ovulation. With the use of a special cannula or a cotton-tipped applicator, the woman obtains daily a little of her vaginal secretion and places it on a glass slide. When the slides are stained and examined microscopically, it is possible to tell very accurately whether ovulation has taken place and the day on which it occurred.

A special urine test for ovulation has also been developed within the last few years. A sample of the woman's urine is obtained daily, and a small amount of it is injected into an immature white rat. Two hours after the urine is injected, the rat is killed and its ovaries are examined. If ovulation had taken place the presence of certain hormones in the woman's urine will cause a congestion of the rat's ovaries, making them appear pinkish or reddish. If no ovulation had occurred, the ovaries retain their usual pale color.

Another method for establishing the occurrence of ovulation is the microscopic examination of a small piece of tissue taken from the lining of the uterus, a procedure known as an endometrial biopsy. This test is usually made just before or on the first day of menstruation. In preparing itself for the reception of the fertilized egg, the lining of the uterus normally undergoes special changes after ovulation has occurred. If it is found that these changes had not taken place, it is presumptive evidence that an ovum did not mature in the ovary that month.

By means of one or the other of these tests, it is now possible to tell with fair accuracy whether ovulation takes place and the day on which it occurs.

If no eggs are produced, would the woman continue to menstruate?

Yes, menstruation may occur without ovulation. The menstrual rhythm may continue quite regularly even though no ova are released. Such cycles are called "anovulatory cycles," and they occur quite frequently during adolescence and prior to the menopause. They may, however, also occur from time to time during the active reproductive period of a woman and be a cause of diminished fertility.

Assuming that a normal egg is produced, is it possible to tell whether the husband's sperm cells actually go up to meet it?

Only indirectly. When ovulation is normal, there is still the possibility that conditions in the genital tract of the wife may interfere with the entrance or passage of the sperm. Such conditions may be present in either the vagina, the cervix or the Fallopian tubes. In cases of infertility, it is therefore necessary to determine whether these channels are open or not.

There are instances, for example, in which the semen cannot be deposited in the vaginal canal because of a tightening of the muscles around the entrance to the vagina which prevents penetration. We shall discuss this condition at another time, but I want to mention it now as a possible cause of infertility.

Once the seminal fluid enters the vagina, what can keep the sperm from going farther up into the womb and the tubes?

Well, obstructions at the opening of the cervix may keep the sperm from entering the uterus. If, for instance, the opening is filled with a thick, tenacious mucous secretion, or if there is some local infection, it may form a barrier to the passage of the sperm. These become enmeshed in the thick mucus and cannot move upward. If the infection is cleared up, conception is likely to follow. There are other conditions besides infections which may cause a blockage of the cervix and keep the sperm from entering the uterus. Each case must, therefore, be investigated individually.

The Postcoital Test

Is it possible to tell whether the sperm enter the uterus?

To establish whether the sperm enter into the uterus, the so-called "postcoital" test is often used. This test was first described nearly a hundred years ago by the famous gynecologist Marion Sims, but it was later improved and popularized by Max Hühner and is often called the Hühner test or the compatibility test. The wife is examined within several hours after she has had relations with her husband, and some of the secretions from the vagina and the cervix are removed and studied microscopically for the presence of sperm and the quality of their vitality. The test is preferably made around the middle of the woman's cycle—that is, at the presumed time of maximal fertility—and it enables the physician to determine whether the sperm enter the cervix and how long they remain active in the vagina and the uterus. Less frequently performed is a test in which samples of the intra-uterine fluid are obtained and examined for the presence of sperm.

Is there any way of knowing whether the sperm cells enter the tubes from the womb?

No. There is no test which shows whether the sperm have actually entered the tubes or not. The tubes are not accessible to any direct examination, nor can any instrument be passed into them without opening the abdomen. It is, however, possible by means of special procedures to determine whether the tubes are open or not; if they are found to be closed, it is assumed that the sperm cannot pass the point of obstruction and therefore do not reach the egg cell.

How can a doctor tell whether the tubes are open or closed?

By a comparatively simple test. This test was described by Dr. I. C. Rubin over forty years ago, and it has proved of very great value. It consists in the introduction of a gas, carbon dioxide, into the uterus under a certain degree of pressure. As the cavity of the uterus becomes filled, the gas soon makes its way into the tubes, and if one or both of them are open it passes through them into the abdomen. If they are closed, the gas cannot pass beyond the point of obstruction. The degree of pressure required to force the gas through, the bubbling sounds which can be heard by listening over the abdomen, the shoulder pains which the woman feels when she sits up afterward, as the gas rises and irritates the diaphragm, and, if necessary, a subsequent X-ray examination tell whether the tubes are open. Various degrees of tubal obstruction can be determined by the amount of pressure required to make the gas pass through. Instead of the gas, a fluid opaque to X rays is sometimes injected into the uterus and the tubes, and X-ray photographs are taken. By this method the condition of the tubes can be studied even more thoroughly.

I might also mention that in addition to the diagnostic value of these tests, the mere passage of the gas or the radio-opaque liquid many times may serve to open a previously obstructed canal and thus aid in the treatment of the infertility.

What causes blocking of the Fallopian tubes, Doctor?

Tubal obstruction is usually the result of some inflammation which leads to a closure of the canal. Among the more frequent sources of such inflammations are gonorrhea, infections following abortion —especially, induced abortion—or childbirth, and, more rarely, tuberculosis. Among other causes which may lead to tubal closure are congenital malformations, growths inside or outside the genital tract, and even muscular spasms which are due to emotional disturbances and anxieties.

Psychological Causes of Infertility

Can sterility be due to emotional disturbances or psychological factors alone?

In many childless couples even thorough diagnostic studies fail to show any physical abnormality. In some of these cases pathological factors are probably present which as yet we have no way of determining; in others, the infertility may possibly be due to psychological disturbances. It is fairly well accepted today that fears, anxieties, and other emotional factors may affect bodily functions, including the reproductive processes. They may influence the ripening of the eggs; they may cause spasms in the Fallopian tubes or other genital passages; or they may interfere with the attachment of the fertilized egg to the wall of the uterus. You have probably heard of women who had been sterile for many years and then became pregnant soon after the couple had adopted a baby. In these cases the infertility may perhaps have been due to emotional conflicts. It is possible that overanxiety about the childlessness may in itself be a factor in infertility.

Is failure of the egg to attach itself to the uterus a frequent cause of infertility?

It is believed now that failure of the fertilized egg to implant itself adequately occurs quite often among infertile couples. The seminal fluid and the ovum may be normal and the genital passages of both the husband and the wife unobstructed, but if the fertilized egg fails to imbed itself in the lining of the uterus no pregnancy will follow.

Such failure may be due to certain hormonal deficiencies or other causes which prevent the lining of the uterus from preparing itself adequately for the reception of the fertilized egg.

The Rh Factor
What about the Rh factor? What role does it play in childlessness?

As I have already mentioned, approximately eighty-five per cent of our white population are Rh positive—that is, they have the Rh factor in their blood—and fifteen per cent are Rh negative. Incompatibilities arise only when an Rh-positive man marries a woman who is Rh negative. Under such circumstances, their child is likely to inherit the Rh-positive blood of the father. As the baby develops in the uterus of the Rh-negative mother, the two bloods will be incompatible, with the result that the child may be born with a destructive blood condition which is technically known as erythroblastosis. This, however, rarely happens with the first or even the second child, and even in later children the incidence of the disturbance is not high.

Treating Infertility
What are the chances for a childless couple to have a baby?

The results of treating an infertile couple may vary from doctor to doctor or from clinic to clinic; they also depend on the nature of the problem. In a group of young couples under thirty years of age who have been trying unsuccessfully to conceive for a year or longer, properly studied and treated, we can expect that more than forty per cent will conceive. Of course, not every clinic can report such results, mainly because most of the couples they treat have already been studied and unsuccessfully treated elsewhere; consequently, most of the specialized centers report a lower percentage of success. The recognition that the male spouse should be studied and the progress made in the evaluation and treatment of the male problem have added to the improvement of the results obtained.

Even more progress has been made in the study and treatment of the female factor. Advances in the diagnosis and handling of some endocrine problems have greatly improved the picture. In the last few years, we have learned about some suprarenal problems that suppress ovulation and how to deal with them. Recently a synthetic compound, as well as extracts from the urine of menopausal women and from human pituitary glands, has been used experimentally to cope with the problem of failure to ovulate.

There has been much publicity about multiple pregnancies in some women treated with these compounds. As we learn more about diagnosis of the situation producing lack of ovulation and also about adequate management of these drugs, we may expect to be able to solve medical problems which until now have been absolutely insoluble.

Artificial Insemination

What is artificial insemination? Is it what the newspapers refer to as "test-tube babies"?

Artificial insemination means the artificial or mechanical introduction of male seminal fluid into the female genital tract for the purpose of inducing impregnation. The only artificial element in this procedure is the mechanical injection of the seminal fluid by a doctor. The sperm are still the sperm of the man, and the egg must, of course, be the egg of the woman; and conception will occur only when the two meet in the woman's Fallopian tube, and not in a laboratory test tube.

Is this a recent development in medicine?

No. Artificial insemination has been practiced for a long time, but at first only on animals. The first recorded experiment of an artificial impregnation was made in 1784 by the Italian scientist Spallanzani. In his *Dissertations,* he tells how he confined a female dog in a room and later, when she showed evidence of being "in heat," obtained a small amount of seminal fluid from a male dog of the same breed and injected it through a syringe into the vagina and the uterus of the female. Sixty-two days later she brought forth three young ones, who resembled in color and shape both the mother and the absentee father. After describing the original experiment, Spallanzani very quaintly adds—here is his statement—"Thus did I succeed in fecundating this quadruped; and I can truly say that I never received greater pleasure upon any occasion, since I first cultivated experimental philosophy."

Since then this type of "experimental philosophy" has been practiced extensively on a variety of animals, including almost all the laboratory animals, from the sea urchin to the monkey. Artificial insemination is widely performed also on a wide variety of animals bred for commercial purposes, such as bees, chickens, turkeys, horses, sheep, cows and pigs. The success of this procedure is such that artificially inseminated cows produce calves equal to those born of cows that have been mated naturally.

What is the object of artificial insemination of animals? Is it performed only for experimental purposes?

No. Artificial insemination of animals is now usually performed for economic reasons and for the purpose of developing better breeds. It is said that the method was used by Arabian horse breeders some six hundred years ago, but it is only since the beginning of the present century that its practical potentialities have become generally recognized. With this method a large number of females can be impregnated with the sperm of a single specially selected male. With proper care, the collected seminal fluid can even be sent over great distances, so the procedure is well adapted for animal breeding. The method is widely employed at the present time both abroad and in this country for the raising of select horses and cattle. Since the semen of stud animals, especially champion animals, is a precious commodity, and since it is so rich in sperm, a single ejaculate is diluted and used for the insemination of many female animals—up to eighty cows in the case of some bulls. The advances made in the preservation of semen by improvement of the diluting fluids and freezing at very low temperatures enable the husbandman to inseminate cows with the semen of choice bulls anywhere in the world successfully up to four years after ejaculation, and perhaps long after the bull is no longer fertile.

Artificial insemination is also employed in cases of animal infertility when, because of some anatomical difficulty, copulation and direct insemination by the male are not possible.

Artificial Insemination of Human Beings

What about women? How long has artificial insemination been used on human beings?

The oldest report of artificial insemination in humans was made by John Hunter, a famous British surgeon, late in the eighteenth century; but it was not until recently that the practice came into more general use. At the present time artificial inseminations of women are resorted to quite frequently for the purpose of overcoming certain types of infertility, the seminal fluid either of the husband or of another male being used, depending upon the conditions. We have already seen that some conditions, such as impotence of the husband, or obstructions at the entrance to the vagina or the cervix, may make it impossible for the sperm to enter the uterus. Under such circumstances it may be advisable to introduce a few drops of the husband's seminal fluid directly into the uterine opening by means of a small syringe, at the time in the woman's cycle when she is most likely to be fertile—that is, around the time of ovulation.

But if the husband is sterile, would an artificial insemination be of any value?

An artificial insemination with the husband's seminal fluid can be successful only when his sperm are fairly normal in quantity and quality. If he has no sperm cells or only a very few in his seminal fluid, the procedure would be of no value. When a man is found to be sterile, the question sometimes comes up of inseminating his wife with the fluid of another male, or donor.

Are artificial inseminations often done with the semen of a man other than the husband?

Yes, this method of overcoming childlessness is now widely practiced when the problem is found to be in the husband and when his condition is not amenable to treatment. When the desire of a couple for offspring is very strong and the choice lies between adoption and an artificial insemination with a donor's fluid, they may prefer the latter, which is sometimes referred to as "semi-adoption" or therapeutic insemination. In this way they can be sure that the child will inherit qualities of a least one of them; both will share the experience of the pregnancy and the birth.

What is generally the attitude of the husband toward such a child?

The husband, even during the period of pregnancy, usually begins to look upon the coming child as his own. The child usually brings great joy to both wife and husband and adds to the stability of the family. I know a number of couples who have had two and even three children by artificial insemination and who are very happy with their families.

I would emphasize the fact, however, that an artificial insemination with a donor's fluid should be undertaken only after careful consideration on the part of the couple and the physician. It should be done only at the mutual desire and with the full consent of both husband and wife. The couple should not know the identity of the donor, nor should the donor know the identity of the recipient. It is essential, of course, that the donor's family and personal medical history be well ascertained and that he be fertile and in good physical and mental health.

Are artificial inseminations usually successful?

This may vary very much, according to the quality of the semen used and the fertility of the woman. When the husband's semen is deficient in numbers or other qualities of the sperm, it might take a number of inseminations before the wife gets pregnant, and in many cases this may be a frustrating and unsuccessful experience.

When donor insemination is resorted to, sometimes—though infrequently—a woman may be impregnated after a single insemination. Usually the procedure has to be repeated over a period of several months before the desired conception results. In a few instances, inseminations are unsuccessful, perhaps because the woman herself may not be fertile.

What about the legality of artificial inseminations?

Differences of opinion exist concerning the legality of the procedure and the legitimacy of the children born as a result of it. The assumption is that when the insemination is undertaken at the request of both husband and wife, the child is naturally theirs and should be considered as if they had voluntarily adopted it. While the question of the legitimacy of the child has not yet been legally established, it would seem to me that the problem of legitimacy hardly comes into consideration when both parents are eager to have a child by this method.

Most parents and doctors prefer to register the child as the natural offspring of both husband and wife; if any reservations are voiced by either of the spouses the doctor would rather not go ahead with the procedure.

If the wife is the one who is permanently sterile, is there any measure of this kind to help the situation?

No, obviously not. It is not yet possible to obtain the egg of a woman, or to implant it artificially. However, apropos of your question, you may be interested in a rather unusual request which I received not long ago. A woman, thirty-five years of age, and very happily married for ten years to a college professor, found that she was permanently sterile. She had even submitted herself to an operation in the hope that her condition could be corrected, but during the operation it was found that she had a congenital abnormality which made impregnation and childbearing impossible. She felt very keenly that it would be unfair to deprive her husband of a child because of her disability, and after months of deliberation and discussion with him she made this proposal—let me quote her words— "Would it be possible to find some woman who would be willing to bear a child by my husband for us? The procedure, I believe, could be carried out in a purely scientific and impersonal manner, by hospitalization and artificial impregnation. I feel that there are women of desirable types who would be glad to provide such service for a reasonable fee." In other words, she was looking not for a donor father, but for a donor mother—for a woman who would be willing to be artificially impregnated with the professor's seminal fluid, bear a child, and then surrender the child to them.

In this connection I might tell you of a very interesting experiment which was performed by two biologists at Harvard. They removed ten egg cells from a female rabbit and fertilized them in the laboratory by bringing them into contact with the semen of a male rabbit. Then they transplanted the fertilized eggs into the Fallopian tube of another female rabbit. These eggs proceeded to develop within the body of the third rabbit, and after thirty-three days seven young rabbits, bearing the coloring and characteristics of their real parents, were born to this "artificial" mother.

Similar experiments have been carried out successfully on cows and other animals. However, no human experiments along this line have been attempted.

Artificial Fertilization

If the eggs and the sperm can be made to unite outside the body, is it then possible to produce a full-grown organism in the laboratory?

Yes, but only in those species in which fertilization and development normally take place outside the female body, as in fish, frogs and other types of aquatic organisms. Here, as we have already seen, the female discharges her eggs to the outside, while the male emits his sperm in the immediate vicinity, and the union of the two sex elements occurs in the surrounding medium. Under such circumstances it is comparatively simple to obtain the female eggs and the male sperm and bring them together in the laboratory or breeding tank. This, in fact, is being done on a rather large scale in the breeding of certain fish for commercial purposes.

However, biologists have gone even a step further, and have shown that in certain species of animals it is actually possible to cause the development of the egg by artificial means without any sperm cells at all.

Parthenogenesis (Virgin Birth)

Do you mean that an egg which has not been fertilized by a sperm can develop into a living organism?

Yes. It has long been recognized that the eggs of certain species of animals are normally capable of developing without fertilization. The queen bee, for instance, lays two types of eggs, fertilized and unfertilized. Both develop into mature bees, except that the unfertilized eggs grow up into males or drones, while those that are fertilized produce workers or queens. The development of eggs without fertilization is known by the rather long name of parthenogenesis, or "virgin birth," and occurs in several species of animals under certain circumstances.

Artificial Parthenogenesis

Several scientists have succeeded in causing eggs which normally require sperm fertilization to develop into new individuals without the intervention of sperm. They have accomplished this by substituting certain physico-chemical stimulants for the fertilizing action of the sperm cells. Thus, Jacques Loeb, the American biologist, found that by adding in a definite sequence various kinds of chemicals to sea water containing the eggs of sea urchins, he could induce the complete development of these eggs into the adult form. Among the substances which were employed as substitutes for male sperm were such prosaic chemicals as salt, alcohol, ether, chloroform and even potassium cyanide. Later it was found that the eggs of frogs could be induced to develop by merely puncturing them with a needle. Loeb treated frogs' eggs in this manner and actually succeeded in raising about half a dozen frogs to the adult stage. These, then, were parthenogenetic, or virgin-born frogs, produced from eggs without the aid of any male element, and they could in no way be distinguished from frogs which develop in the normal manner through fertilization with sperm. Strangely enough, all the virgin-born frogs proved to be males. However, in the case of most animals, especially mammals, including man, such offspring would always be females.

The fact that an ovum can develop without fertilization would indicate that, at least in the lower forms of life, the potentialities for developing new organisms are inherent in the egg itself. The ovum is like a wound-up mechanism, ready to start unfolding under the proper stimulus, and this stimulus may be supplied either by a sperm cell or by other physico-chemical means.

In regard to man, from time to time we hear reports of successful fertilization and development to the stage of a few cells in the laboratory. However, up to the present most serious investigators question whether successful fertilization of a human egg and development to a few cells has ever been accomplished.

These are certainly fascinating experiments. They remind me of the fantasy in Shaw's Back to Methuselah, *in which a human child is incubated in an egg outside the mother's body. Maybe someday reproduction will really take place in the laboratory.*

Perhaps. You will find, incidentally, that the British scientist Haldane went even farther than Shaw in such fantasies. In his imaginative booklet on the future of science, *Daedalus,* he envisioned a time when the majority of human children will be born in the laboratory, or "ectogenetically," as he termed it. The ovary of a woman would be removed at puberty and kept in a suitable medium, and as the eggs matured each month they would be artificially fertilized with sperm. The resulting embryos would be incubated in the laboratory for nine months and then brought out into the world. Naturally, only the sex cells of the most eugenically suitable men and women would be selected for breeding purposes.

As a matter of fact, when specimens of human semen are placed in glass tubes and frozen instantaneously, the sperm do not lose their vitality for a long time. Even after remaining in a frozen state for many months, a good proportion of the sperm cells regain their motility when the semen is thawed out. With improved techniques it is quite likely that it will be possible to keep the sperm in a dormant condition for almost any length of time. Such possibilities open up new vistas for biological investigation in the field of human fertility.

H. J. Muller, the American biologist, in his booklet *Out of the Night,* has even suggested that eventually the sperm of selected men might be kept alive in some way long after the death of the individuals, and be used in artificial inseminations for the eugenic improvement of mankind. Thus a man might become the father of numerous offspring long after he himself had been gathered unto his ancestors. The problem, of course, might still remain as to who the supermen should be whose seminal fluids would be saved for such purposes. These considerations, however, are but scientific fancies, and for the present we must still content ourselves with the old-fashioned, well proved and enjoyable mode of having children.

Miscarriages and Abortions

Is it true that the risk of miscarriage is greater in women who have had difficulty conceiving?

Yes. Of the conceptions occurring among infertile couples, a large proportion—larger than for the general population—terminate in a miscarriage, or spontaneous abortion, as it would be more correct to say. You may be interested to know that for all the mammals studied, nearly a third of all conceptions result in spontaneous abortion or pregnancy wastage. The same is probably true for humans. Many of these occur so early in the pregnancy that the woman does not even realize that she is pregnant. Others go on for a few months and, for a variety of reasons, such as poor development of the egg, genetic defects, endocrine problems of the mother, poor development and functioning of the placenta, intercurrent disease, etc., may be spontaneously terminated. This constitutes a very serious medical problem.

What is the difference between a miscarriage and an abortion?

Both imply a premature termination or interruption of a pregnancy. Technically there is a distinction between the two words according to whether the pregnancy ends in the early or later months. In ordinary usage, however, the term "miscarriage" is applied to a spontaneous and involuntary ending of a pregnancy at any time before the seventh month, while "abortion" is used to indicate an artificial and deliberate interruption of a pregnancy. When a pregnancy terminates after the seventh month, but before full term—that is, at a time when the baby is generally large enough to have a fair chance for survival—it is called a premature birth. However, as I stated before, doctors in general prefer to call all involuntary pregnancy terminations spontaneous abortions.

The Causes of Miscarriages

Why do women miscarry?

The causes of miscarriages are quite complex, and many of them are not yet fully understood. Generally speaking, a miscarriage may result because the fertilized egg is in some way defective and lacks sufficient vitality to develop completely, or else because certain deficiencies or abnormalities in the mother lead to untimely uterine contractions which expel the fetus. Perhaps seventy per cent of all miscarriages are due to defects in the embryo itself, caused either by abnormalities in the egg or the sperm or by factors connected with the early development of the fertilized egg. Under such circumstances, the normal growth and development of the embryo cannot continue, and the miscarriage, therefore, may in reality prevent the birth of defective offspring.

Among the maternal factors which may lead to the premature expulsion of the fetus are such conditions as growths in and around the uterus, displacements of the uterus, glandular disturbances, vitamin deficiencies, local or general infections, and premature dilation of the neck of the womb. Emotional disturbances too may be responsible for miscarriages in some instances. There is also evidence that blood incompatibilities between the mother and the developing baby may possibly lead to the death of the fetus in the early months of pregnancy. Nearly three fourths of all miscarriages, incidentally, occur before the fourth month.

Prevention of Miscarriages

Are there any measures that can be taken to prevent a miscarriage?

The better the physical condition of a woman at the time she conceives, the more likely she is to go through her pregnancy with little difficulty. It is advisable, therefore, to have a thorough preconceptional examination, so that whatever abnormalities may be present can be corrected in time. During pregnancy it is always advisable for a woman to place herself under the care of her family physician or obstetrician, who will supervise her prenatal period and treat any difficulty that may arise.

Even when there is a threatened abortion, measures can still be taken to prevent it. The actual onset of a spontaneous abortion is usually preceded by forewarning symptoms such as vaginal discharge of a bloodstained fluid or bearing-down pains in the lower abdomen and back. Suitable medical care may at this point prevent the interruption of the pregnancy.

Does staining in the early months of pregnancy always mean the beginning of a miscarriage?

No. The mere appearance of a bloodstained discharge does not necessarily indicate a threatened miscarriage. As a matter of fact, nearly one third of all pregnant women experience some staining or bleeding in the early months, yet the majority of them continue with a normal pregnancy. While the occurrence of bleeding does not necessarily indicate the onset of an abortion, nevertheless any genital bleeding or staining during a pregnancy should be immediately investigated.

If a woman has had one spontaneous abortion, does it mean that she is more likely to miscarry again in future pregnancies?

The majority of spontaneous abortions result from factors which are not likely to recur in subsequent pregnancies. Only a very small percentage of women who miscarry show a habitual tendency in this direction. If a woman has had one miscarriage, however, she should have a thorough examination before she plans her next pregnancy, and careful supervision throughout the period of gestation. In this way any preventive or corrective measures that may become necessary could be undertaken in time.

A neighbor of ours who was three months pregnant fell down several steps and miscarried a few days later. Are accidents of this kind apt to produce a miscarriage?

There is a rather widespread, though much exaggerated, fear that some slight accident during pregnancy might result in a miscarriage. Some women, it is true, are especially sensitive and are apt to miscarry as a result of some minor physical or emotional shock. As a rule, however, even violent exercise and severe strains do not influence the progress of a normal pregnancy.

Stillbirths

Why are some babies born dead even though they have been carried the full nine months?

When a child is dead at birth, it is known as a stillbirth. In the

United States, according to the latest data available, there are 16.2 stillbirths for every thousand babies born alive. The causes responsible for this high stillbirth rate are still not fully understood. Considerable medical attention is now being given to studies of the factors involved and of the measures that can be taken to reduce the stillbirth rate.

Bibliography

Amelar, R. D., *Infertility in Men*. Davis, 1966.

Bassett, William T., *Counseling the Childless Couple*. Prentice-Hall, 1963.

Finegold, Wilfred J., M.D., *Artificial Insemination*. Thomas, 1964.

Gebhard, P. H., Pomeroy, W. B., Martin, C. E., and Christenson, C. V., *Pregnancy, Birth and Abortion*. Science Editions paperback (Wiley), 1966.

Guttmacher, Alan F., M.D., *The Consumers Union Report on Family Planning*, 2nd ed. Consumers Union of the U.S., 1966.

Hamblen, Edwin C., *Facts for Childless Couples*, 2nd ed. Thomas, 1960.

Isaac, Rael Jean, *Adopting a Child Today*. Harper and Row, 1965.

Kleegman, Sophie J., and Kaufman, S. A., *Infertility in Women*. Davis, 1966.

Lader, Lawrence, *Abortion*. Bobbs-Merrill, 1966.

Portnoy, Louise, and Saltman, Jules, *Fertility in Marriage: A Guide for the Childless*. Collier paperback, 1962.

St. John-Stevas, Norman, *Right to Life*. Holt, Rinehart and Winston, 1964.

Stone, Abraham, M.D., "How Can We Have A Baby?," *Redbook* Magazine, May 1954.

CHAPTER VII

THE ART OF MARRIAGE

Until now we have concerned ourselves mainly with the biological aspects of marriage and reproduction. Today I should like to consider with you briefly the sex side of marriage—the physical, psychological and emotional factors involved in the sex relation. Within recent years it has become more generally recognized that sex plays a dominant role in marriage, and that a satisfactory sex relationship is essential for a happy union. What is perhaps less frequently appreciated is the fact that a harmonious and dynamic sex adjustment does not necessarily develop spontaneously, but requires an understanding of the nature and the mechanism of the sex union as well as the exercise of an art in sexual love.

Marriage and Sex

Isn't there a tendency at present to stress the sex side of marriage too much? From some of the discussions on the subject I get the impression at times that sex is considered almost the only purpose and the only basis of marriage.

I quite agree with you that sex alone does not make a marriage, and that no really lasting relationship can be based merely on sexual attraction. For a happy marriage, there must of course be present mutual love and affection, a community of ideas, of interests, of tastes, of standards, an adequate economic arrangement and a satisfactory adjustment in personal, family, and social relationships. On the other hand, it is also true that a successful marriage can hardly be achieved where sexual attraction does not exist, or where the marital sex life is unsatisfactory. In our work we have constantly found that many domestic difficulties can be traced directly or indirectly to sexual disharmonies, and that the sex factor plays a leading role in marital satisfaction. A number of studies in recent years have also emphasized this fact. Dickinson and Beam, for instance, in a summary of their analytical survey of a thousand marriages state as follows: "If the data in this study reinforce any one concept it is that satisfactory sexual relations are necessary to fully adjusted and successful unions."

The Ethics of Sex

Isn't it true, though, that the constant emphasis on sex tends to put the marital relation on a mere physical level and destroys some of the ideals of marriage?

Unfortunately, not all of our present marriage ideals lead to an ideal marriage. The very disposition, which still exists, to regard the sexual embrace as essentially sinful, impure and degrading is a serious deterrent to a satisfactory marital life. In a wise discussion of marriage and the ethics of sex, John Haynes Holmes, minister of the Community Church in New York, once said—but let me quote his words—

How many men and women there are—not as many today as there were yesterday, but millions of them still—who believe that there is something wrong about the sex life! How many husbands and wives there are who have entered upon their relationship together with the secret conviction that what they are doing is something to be ashamed of and hidden away. How many wives there are who cherish the suspicion, never to be reached by any argument or logic, that their practice of sex is an ignoble yielding to the flesh, and who have never surrendered to their husbands except with feelings of protest and humiliation! I know of nothing so disastrous to happiness in marriage as this feeling of shame which is so often attached to what possesses us with so insistent a drive upon our energies.

It would be well indeed, it seems to me, if we were to cease to look upon the sex urge as one of our "baser" instincts and as an unworthy motive in matrimony. If anything, the development of a harmonious sex life should constitute one of the aims and ideals of the marital union.

It happens, of course, that in the transition from the prudishness and false modesties of former generations, some lean too far in the opposite direction. We must remember, however, that we are only now emerging from the puritanical era with its taboos and inhibitions, and that any undue emphasis on sex and sexual technique at the present time may well be only a reaction to the suppressions and repressions of the previous age.

What has led to the present-day change in attitude toward sex values generally? More, it seems to me, is being written about sex today than ever before.

Many social and cultural factors have undoubtedly combined to bring about a newer attitude toward sex. The growing emancipation and independence of women have enabled them to exercise greater freedom and initiative in the choice of a mate and in the expression of their sexual desires. The spread of birth-control knowledge has made possible the separation of sex from reproduction and the realization of a more dynamic sex expression in marriage. The rise of Freudian psychology with its emphasis upon the libido, and the wider dissemination of books on sex questions—the books of Havelock Ellis, Margaret Sanger, Marie Stopes, Van de Velde, Dickinson, Kinsey, Masters and Johnson, and others—have brought about an increased awareness of the significance of the sexual impulse, and have centered greater attention upon the importance of the sexual side of marriage. At the same time, the widespread and rapid industrial, economic, political, and cultural changes of our age, by giving rise to new social values, have forced a re-evaluation and reappraisal of our former sexual attitudes, ethics and standards.

As for the problems of sexual technique, the recognition that some preparation is necessary for sexual love is not at all a modern discovery. Among primitive groups guidance in sexual matters is regularly given to young people by their elders, often constituting a part of the initiation ceremonies at puberty. Malinowski, for instance, reports that the boys and girls of the Trobriand Islands receive routine instruction in erotic matters from their elders and companions. Among the Samoans too, according to Margaret Mead, definite information concerning the details of sex life is generally imparted to young people, and "the need of a technique to deal with sex as an art" is fully recognized among them. As far as civilized peoples are concerned, books on the art of sex have been written long before our present era. The manner of wooing and the art of sex were dealt with in an Egyptian papyrus which dates back some three thousand years; they were described in great detail in the Hindu *Kama Sutra,* written about sixteen hundred years ago; in the poems of Ovid, who lived during the first century, and who, in fact, originated the term "art of love"; in the *Perfumed Garden* of Arabia, written in the sixteenth century; and in many other ancient books. It is only in the last few centuries that the art of sex has been largely neglected and even suppressed. Now we are once again realizing the importance of an understanding approach in sexual love, and are placing greater emphasis upon an adequate and varied technique in the marital sex relation.

The Sex Instinct

Why should there be a need, though, for so much discussion about the details of the art of love? Aren't the natural human instincts and impulses a sufficient guide to a satisfactory sex life?

Well, neither in our social sex conduct nor in our individual sex behavior can we rely entirely upon our instincts. Generally speaking, an instinct is an innate tendency to behave in a specific manner when confronted by a certain stimulus. In civilized human life, however, we long ago ceased to respond in an instinctive manner to sexual stimuli. From early infancy our sex impulses are subjected to restriction, suppressions and taboos which effectively modify our normal sex instincts and condition us against a natural sex expression. These inhibitions are not easily thrown off even after wedlock, and the development of an adequate sex life in marriage cannot, therefore, be "left to nature" altogether. It requires a conscious and intelligent effort for its realization.

Furthermore, it is a significant biological fact that the sexual urge of men and women is in itself not sufficient to guide them to a satisfactory physical union. The word "instinct" implies the ability to act in a certain manner without previous education in the performance. In the human species, however, the actual technique of sex is predominantly a learned process. Without some previous knowledge and understanding of the mechanism of coitus, difficulties in the sexual union are very apt to occur. Let me quote to you an interesting passage on this topic from an article by Parshley, author of *The Science of Human Reproduction:*

> In most mammals . . . copulatory behavior is instinctive, being not at all dependent upon imitation, learning or experience. Experiments show that individuals reared to maturity in isolation can at once perform the act, if the mate is presented when in proper physiological condition. . . . In contrast complete copulatory behavior among the primates (that is, among monkeys, apes and men) is reached only after a long period of experimentation and experience. It is not an instinctive behavior pattern, but rather a complex adjustment between two individuals, made possible through early training and facilitated by more or less prolonged association.

In other words, adequate copulatory behavior does not come instinctively to men and women. The technique of the sexual relation has to be learned in order to develop a satisfactory sex life.

Sex Technique

What specifically do you mean by "sexual technique"? What particular knowledge does it require?

When I speak of the technique of sex, I am referring to the effective performance of the sexual act. This requires, first of all, an understanding of the mechanism involved, of the anatomical and physiological processes of sexual union; and second, an appreciation of the art of sexual love—that is, of the means by which the sex relationship may be made most satisfying to both mates.

From a physical viewpoint, the sex act involves the union or coaptation of the male and female genitals. It is well that both the man and the woman should have some understanding of the structure and functions of the sex organs, their respective relations to each other, the changes which occur during sexual stimulation and excitation, the position to be taken in order to bring the organs into satisfactory apposition—in other words, the actual mechanism of the sexual union. It may not be necessary to follow Balzac's rhetorical suggestion that a man should not marry "before he has studied anatomy and has dissected at least one woman," but it is certainly true that some knowledge of sexual anatomy is of considerable help to the satisfactory consummation of the sex act.

On the psychological and emotional side, it is desirable that the couple should know something about the nature of the sexual impulse, the stimuli which lead to sexual excitation, the differences in the sexual responses and reactions between the male and the female, and the value and importance of a delicacy, finesse, and skill in the sexual approach.

The Nature of the Sex Act

Are there special changes that occur during sexual stimulation, Doctor?

Nearly every part of the body is brought into activity during sexual stimulation and sexual union. The nervous mechanism, the glandular system, the muscular apparatus, the special senses, particularly the senses of touch, of sight, of odor—all of them play a part in sex activity. The physical changes which take place during the sexual relations are, in fact, so widespread that they involve the entire organism.

The physical act itself consists of the insertion of the male organ into the vaginal passage of the female, and of the reciprocal copulatory movements which lead to the climax, or orgasm. Under ordinary conditions the penis is soft and flaccid, but during sexual excitement it becomes firm, erect and sufficiently rigid to penetrate into the vagina. The female genitals, too, undergo certain changes upon sexual arousal. The walls of the vagina become congested, the vaginal opening relaxes and even pouts to some extent, and the clitoris and the smaller labiae become tense and slightly erect. At the same time the glands of the vulva secrete a slippery fluid which moistens the surfaces of the external genitals and helps the entry of the penis. Accompanying the local changes there are general physical and emotional manifestations of sexual stimulation—the stronger and quicker pulse, the faster breathing, the dilated pupils, the flushed face, the increased muscular activity and nervous excitation. The coital movements increasingly heighten the erotic sensations and the rising tension until the release is reached in the orgasm.

The Defloration

Is the first sex act actually very painful for the woman?

Not necessarily. The first or first few sexual relations differ from the subsequent acts in that the hymen is penetrated at this time. Any pain experienced is due to the actual stretching or breaking of the hymen, and the degree of discomfort depends largely upon the texture and condition of this membrane. If it is thin and elastic it will dilate or give way with but little discomfort; if it is firm and tense, it may prove to be quite resistant, and entry will then cause considerable pain. Even this, however, can be greatly lessened, if not entirely avoided, by an understanding and patient approach by the husband, as well as by the cooperation and relaxation of the wife.

Is the hymen always broken during the first sex act?

Unless the hymen was previously stretched by other means, it is broken at this time, if complete penetration takes place. The hymen partially surrounds the vaginal entrance, and the male organ must pass through it in order to enter the vaginal canal. The diameter of the erect penis is about an inch and a half, while that of the opening through the hymen is generally about an inch. The pressure of the male organ first causes the hymen to stretch or dilate, and if this is not sufficient to permit entry, the continued pressure results in the breaking of the membrane at one or more points. This constitutes the defloration.

How much bleeding usually occurs when the hymen is broken? Does it require any particular treatment at the time?

As a rule the bleeding is slight and rarely requires any special treatment. It usually stops in a short time, though there may be a slight recurrence during the first few subsequent relations.

If the first experiences prove uncomfortable, is it advisable to postpone sex relations for a time?

In the *Kama Sutra,* a Hindu classic on marital conduct, Vatsyayana gives the advice that a husband should take ten days in gradually gaining the confidence of his wife before even attempting to consummate the marital union. I doubt whether this counsel is either suitable or necessary for the modern couple, who have probably already had a long period of courtship. It is usually best for the sexual union to be consummated during the first few days after marriage, if feasible. If the attempt at entry should prove to be very painful, or if there is much apprehension and fear on the part of the wife, complete penetration need not take place during the first sex act. A gradual and gentle dilatation carried out during the several successive relationships will considerably ease the discomfort and lessen the anxiety for the woman.

In general, however, even if the first experiences prove uncomfortable, it is not advisable to put off the consummation of the sex union for any length of time. The longer this is postponed the greater will be the feeling of anxiety on the part of the wife and of frustration on the part of the husband. When the completion of the sex union is avoided from day to day under one pretext or another, it is usually a sign of some physiological or emotional difficulty, and if such a situation persists, it is wise to seek medical advice.

Is it true that the first sex experiences have an important bearing upon later adjustment in marriage? I have heard that sexual troubles at the beginning may have a lasting effect on a couple's marital relations.

The importance of the experiences on the so-called "bridal night," as far as future marital happiness is concerned, has been rather exaggerated. It is quite true that awkwardness, clumsiness and much discomfort at the beginning may make the future adjustment more difficult. The woman, particularly, may feel keenly disillusioned and upset by such an experience, and she may resent further sexual contacts for a time. It is not, however, the first relations only that count, but rather the attitude and approach toward the sex union through the months and years of marriage that follow. It is well to bear in mind that some difficulty and perhaps even discomfort are very likely to be encountered at the beginning, and that the first sex relations may not be entirely satisfactory. If this happens, however, it should not be especially disappointing. Gradually, with greater understanding and increasing experience, with patience and consideration, a mutually satisfactory sex life can generally be established.

At the beginning of marriage, many women find it difficult to yield to the sexual union, and, because of modesty, or because of their early training and upbringing, or because of an exaggerated fear of the possible discomforts, they may physically resist the sex act. Ordinarily the intimacies during the premarital courtship tend to develop a feeling of confidence and trust on the part of the woman and to lessen her resistance to the sex relation. At times, however, the resistance may persist for a long period after marriage, irrespective of the wife's affections for her husband, or of her desire to respond to the sexual embrace. As a matter of fact, she may feel a very deep attraction for her mate and possess a strong sexual urge, and yet be unable to prevent an unconscious withdrawal from the relationship. This may make the early sex experiences more difficult to consummate, and cause considerable anxiety during the first weeks of marriage. It is well, therefore, for both the man and the woman to recognize this situation, should it arise, and to treat it with the necessary understanding and patience. The woman, in particular, should realize that complete relaxation on her part and an active cooperation are necessary for the consummation of the sexual union.

Primitive Artificial Defloration

I once read that among certain primitive peoples the hymen is artificially removed or broken before marriage.

Yes, this is a rather common practice among some primitive races in various parts of the world. Books on anthropology abound with examples of this custom. Among many peoples the membrane is artificially dilated either at puberty or just before marriage as a tribal ritual. In their classic book *Woman,* Ploss and Bartels state that in certain countries the hymen is even removed early in infancy. This is so, for instance, in parts of China and Japan, where the membrane is unintentionally destroyed by the mother or nurse as a result of the too energetic cleansing of the infant's genitals, and many physicians in these countries are said not even to be aware of the existence of the hymen. The social, emotional and sentimental significance attached to virginity is a comparatively recent development in the evolution of human culture.

Surgical Defloration

Is it advisable to have the hymen stretched by a doctor before marriage? Some of my friends have had this done.

That would depend upon the attitude of the couple and upon the condition of the hymen. A premarital surgical dilatation of the hymen is sometimes of value as an aid to early marital adjustment. It should be considered especially when the hymen is found to be usually thick and resistant, so that much difficulty might be expected from a natural defloration. An office dilatation of the hymen is a comparatively simple procedure and is made practically painless with the use of a local anesthetic. It rarely requires cutting, causes very little bleeding, and does not incapacitate the woman in any way. This step, however, should be taken only with the express knowledge of the fiancé, for many people still have strong traditional, sentimental or other objections to such a procedure.

I should emphasize once more, though, that with a mutually sympathetic and understanding attitude on the part of both the husband and the wife, the first sex relation need not be accompanied by any considerable physical discomfort, and certainly not by any emotional strain.

Is the woman likely to have any pleasurable sensations from the first sexual relations?

She may or she may not. Many women react immediately to sexual contact and derive the usual type of sexual satisfaction from the very beginning of the marital relation. A fairly high percentage of women, however, do not react fully to the sexual embrace until some time after sex relations have been established. In fact, some women even feel a keen sense of disappointment at first. During the period of courtship, with the accompanying intimacies, the young woman may have received much pleasure from the usual sex play, and she expects the sexual relation to prove even more keenly satisfying. When, because of pain, or fear, or inhibitions, or a lack of reaction to vaginal contact, the sex union gives her little pleasure or is even uncomfortable, she is apt to feel very much disillusioned. It is well for the young wife not to be too deeply concerned if the first sex relations do not prove to be all that she expected. It may take weeks, months, and sometimes even longer before completely satisfying reactions and responses are established.

Once sex relations have been consummated, how can a mutually satisfactory sexual adjustment be achieved?

It is well to bear in mind that the sexual union is both a physical and an emotional experience; it combines sensuality and sentiment. To render the sexual embrace most satisfying in marriage, the husband and the wife should make every effort to understand and appreciate each other's reactions and responses, to harmonize their sexual needs, and to cultivate what has been called the "art of sex" in their relationship.

The Art of Sex
But what exactly do you mean by "the art of sex," Doctor?

The art of sex is the harmonious blending of the physical, emotional and aesthetic qualities of the sexual relationship. The sexual embrace should become neither a duty nor a routine of marriage. It should be a shared experience, with husband and wife each attempting to make the relationship mutually pleasing. In his quaint little *Ritual for Married Lovers,* Guyot, a French physician, wrote almost a century ago: "The joy of sex union is peculiar in this, that it is far greater for the man when he feels it in the woman, and for the woman when she feels it in the man." In other words, the joy of sex is greatly increased for both the man and the woman when it is mutual, and an art in sexual love must aim at achieving this harmony.

Isn't it usual, though, for sexual desire and response to be mutual?

Not necessarily. Too often either the husband or the wife will fail to consider the physical and emotional needs of the other. The husband may not appreciate the fact that a woman's sexual desires and responses differ from those of a man and require a more sensitive and delicate approach for their satisfactory expression; while the wife may not understand the sexual reactions or needs of her husband and she may fail to cooperate and participate actively in the sexual embrace.

If a man had sexual experiences before marriage, would that give him the necessary knowledge and understanding of the art of sex?

That would depend upon the nature and extent of those experiences. If they are merely casual, and especially so if they are with prostitutes, they certainly do not provide a suitable preparation for the later associations with one's wife. On the subject of premarital relations with prostitutes, Havelock Ellis, in his *Studies in the Psychology of Sex,* makes the following trenchant observation:

The training and experience which a man receives from a prostitute, even under fairly favorable conditions, scarcely form the right preparation for approaching a woman of his own class who has no intimate erotic experiences. The frequent result is that he is liable to waver between two opposite courses of action, both of them mistaken. On the one hand, he may treat his wife as . . . a novice to be speedily moulded into the sexual shape he is most accustomed to. . . . On the other hand . . . he may go to the opposite extreme of treating her with an exaggerated respect, and so fail either to arouse or to gratify her erotic needs.

To this I might add another significant difference. In a casual sexual relation a man rarely takes into consideration the woman's sexual feelings or responses. He seeks primarily to obtain relief for himself and the satisfaction of his own sexual urge, and he usually does not expect to arouse or gratify the woman. Such contacts do not, therefore, necessarily supply him with an understanding of the differences in sexual needs between men and women, or with an appreciation of a proper sexual approach to his wife, a relationship which has so many emotional and aesthetic implications.

The Sex Impulse in Man and Woman

Are there great differences in the degree or intensity of sexual desire between men and women?

The degree of woman's erotic sensibility has long been a matter of considerable dispute. For a time it was seriously maintained that sex desire was primarily or entirely a masculine attribute and that woman was devoid of sexual feelings. Acton, an English physician who was considered an authority on sex matters some seventy years ago, wrote that "the majority of women, happily for society, are not much troubled with sexual feelings," and that the supposition that women possessed any erotic desires was a "vile aspersion." Other writers of that period maintained a similar point of view. Today, with our fuller knowledge of the nature of the sexual impulse, such assumptions are, of course, regarded as baseless. It is true that lack of sexual desire, or frigidity, is met with much more frequently in women than in men, but this does not necessarily indicate an inherent absence of an erotic urge. Early training and the social mores often suppress the normal sex desire in women so that it does not manifest itself so readily in later life. Intrinsically, however, a woman's sexual desires may be just as strong as those of a man.

In what ways do the sexual reactions of men and women differ?

In practically all species the male is sexually the more aggressive and active, while the female is primarily receptive and passive. This difference is expressed even in the very character of the respective sex cells. The sperm is active, restless, constantly in motion, while the egg is quiescent, immobile, waiting, so to speak, for the coming of the sperm. Perhaps in this striking difference in the character of the reproductive cells one sees a counterpart of the profound psychic and emotional difference between the two sexes. At any rate, man's sexual impulse is more active, more easily aroused, and his erotic desires are directed more specifically toward sexual consummation. The woman, on the other hand, is sexually more passive, her desires are aroused more slowly, and they express themselves at first in an urge for general bodily contact and sexual play. Only after a certain degree of erotic excitation is the woman prepared for the consummation of the sexual act. In general, sentiment and emotion play a much more significant role in the sexual reactions and responses of the woman than in those of the man.

In the woman, furthermore, there is a distinct rhythm in the intensity of the sex urge, with a periodic rising and waning during the menstrual month. Spontaneous arousal is not as frequent as in the male, and it is related more or less closely to the cycle of her hormonal output.

Another important difference between the sex reactions of the man and those of the woman is the time element involved in reaching the climax, or orgasm, during intercourse. In the man the entire sexual cycle is much shorter; he is more easily aroused and, unless he specifically restrains himself, he is capable of reaching the climax in a comparatively short period. The woman takes a longer time to become stimulated and also a longer period to reach the orgasm. Her sexual reactions are more diffuse and more variable than those of the male.

The Prelude to the Sex Act

Can the difference in the time element be adjusted, then, if it takes the woman so much longer to be aroused?

With an understanding attitude, mutual sympathy, a conscious effort, and deliberate restraint, an adequate adjustment can usually be established. To make the sex relation a mutually satisfying experience, the woman's erotic impulses should first be so aroused that she desires the consummation of the union. As I mentioned, spontaneous sex desire generally occurs less frequently in the woman than in the man, and it therefore often becomes necessary for the husband to evoke desire in his wife if she is to become receptive to the sexual embrace.

The woman usually requires a period of courtship, of wooing, of caressing, of love play, of bodily contact and erotic manipulation before she is physically ready for the sex act. The husband, as Ambroise Paré, a renowned French surgeon of the sixteenth century, wrote, "when lying with his companion and wife must fondle, caress, pleasurably excite and arouse her emotions if he finds her unready in response." This does not imply, or should not imply, merely a physical stimulation, but rather an attitude, an approach, a prelude which would place the wife in a receptive mood for sex union.

As a matter of fact, there seems to exist a biological need for this preliminary courtship and foreplay. A certain amount of wooing and play prior to sex union has been observed in many forms of animal life. Among animals intercourse is not possible unless the female willingly receives the mate, and the male, as a rule, has to pursue and win the female before she will accept him sexually. It is only in the primates, the apes and human beings, that sexual relations may occur even when the female has no desire for the act. It must be obvious, though, that for a fully adjusted and satisfactory sex life in marriage, the sex act should be made mutually desirable. Balzac once wrote that "a man must never permit himself the pleasure with his wife which he has not the skill to make her desire." In other words, the sexual union should be preceded by wooing and love play to arouse the wife to desire the sexual union.

Sex Play and Sex Arousal

What should the prelude to the sexual act include?

In sexual relations emotional and physical factors are intimately bound together, and the prelude to sexual union should take both these aspects into consideration. On the emotional side, the actual manner of wooing will depend upon the cultural background, the individual sensibility and the temperament of the mates, as well as upon the mood and general circumstances of the moment. Obviously, numberless variations are possible. An approach which may prove highly stimulating to one person at one time may be quite repellent at another time or to another individual. Sometimes a word, a gesture, an allusion, an odor is more effective than prolonged erotic play. It is neither possible nor desirable to prescribe any routine form of behavior or any set rules to be followed. In this intimate sphere of human relations, dependence must be placed largely upon individual spontaneity and skill, as well as upon a mutual understanding and adaptation.

A sensitive emotional approach may be sufficient to arouse a high degree of sexual desire, yet in most instances it is also well to employ direct physical stimulation prior to the actual union. This consists largely of the touch, the caress, the kiss. Unlike the male, in whom the sexually excitable areas are more or less localized, the erogenous zones of the woman are extensive and diffuse. Under favorable emotional circumstances, contact with any part of the body may, in fact, be productive of sexual excitation. Mantegazza once described sexual love as a higher form of tactile sensation. The lips, the neck, the lobes of the ears, the breasts, particularly the nipples, are especially sensitive, and the caress or kiss of these parts will often give rise to strong erotic desires. In the early period of marriage the woman may even be more responsive to general bodily stimulation than to direct genital contact. Only after her natural shyness and reserve have gradually been thrown off is the direct contact with the genital region sexually stimulating. The entire vulvar area is erotically sensitive, and the gentle stroking of the labiae minorae, of the entrance to the vagina, and especially of the clitoris, is highly stimulating to the responsive woman. These organs, as well as the nipples, are supplied with erectile tissue and become more firm and erect under sexual excitation. Special care must be taken, however, that these contacts be gentle and delicate, and that they be carried out only in the presence of moisture. Undue pressure and rough manipulation, especially when the surface is dry, may give rise to unpleasant reactions. Gentle stimulation, on the other hand, may quickly result in a responsiveness of the entire body and readiness for sexual union.

Is it necessary that all of these preliminaries precede every act of intercourse?

That would depend entirely upon individual inclinations, desires and reactions at the time. I would say that any of these measures might be used whenever it becomes advisable to increase the erotic excitability and pleasure of the woman and to bring her to a state of tumescence or sexual readiness. At a time when she has much spontaneous desire she may require little or no precoital stimulation, while at other times she may need considerable preliminary arousal. The character, degree, rhythm and duration of the foreplay will depend upon many factors, but especially upon the rapidity or slowness of the wife's reactions and upon the length of time that the husband is able to maintain an erection before ejaculation. It is largely a question of individual conditions, insight and discernment. The wife, however, should feel free to indicate to her husband the areas of her body that are sexually most sensitive, as well as the type, degree and duration of the stimulation which she may require.

In some of the books I shall mention you will find detailed descriptions of the art of erotic love. You will read of the odors which are intended to arouse sexual desire, of the many types of stimulation suitable for the purpose, of the erotic kiss and the tongue kiss, of the love bite and the genital kiss, of any number of bodily manipulations which may be employed to increase sexual desire and pleasure. The chief value of these descriptions, in my opinion, is that they help to remove inhibitions and fears from the sphere of sexual behavior and to show that there is nothing abnormal in any type of love play. Variations in the sexual approach appear to be a part of the biological pattern of the species to which man belongs, and I believe that no form of sex play is wrong in itself, unless it gives rise to physical injury or to undesirable emotional or aesthetic reactions. It is doubtful, however, whether it is at all advisable to become book-conscious in this respect or to follow any particular routine in the art of sex. One should preferably develop one's own ingenuity and skill, and make sex life a mutual adventure, rather than be guided in every detail by the instructions of a Baedeker in the art of love.

It seems to me that to follow any set rules would remove all spontaneity from the sexual relation.

Quite so, and this is what sometimes actually happens when people try to follow too literally the specific instructions to be found in some books on erotic love. Time and again women have told me that after having read certain passages on the art of sex, their husbands would endeavor to carry out in detail the given directions, with the result that the marital relation would become altogether too artificial and strained a procedure, making it difficult for either of them to relax fully. It is much better to give fuller expression to one's own imagination and inclinations in the pursuit of a satisfactory sexual adjustment.

In this connection I should also like to emphasize that during the intimate contacts of sex life, the wife need not and should not be passive. It may be quite true that a woman often prefers to be persuaded or even forced to do the thing that she may very much desire herself, yet it is a serious error for her to remain entirely inactive and inert during sex play. Nothing will dampen the desires of even an ardent husband more completely than actual or feigned sexual indifference on the part of the wife. This is a frequent source of marital disharmony which I intend to discuss with you more fully later. At the beginning of their sex life many women are naturally diffident and timid in their behavior, and the husband must assume all the initiative, but after complete intimacy has been established it is well that the wife too take an active part in the love play and at times initiate the sex relation. It is neither abnormal nor degrading for the woman to make use of all the erotic plays that a man does. For, just as the husband's attempts to stimulate his wife serve at the same time to arouse and increase his own tumescence and desire, so does active participation on the part of the woman excite her own erotic desires and prepare her more fully for the sexual union and responses.

Can a husband tell when his wife has been sufficiently aroused and is ready for sexual union?

Yes, he can often learn to recognize the emotional and physical signs of the degree of the wife's arousal. Where there is mutual frankness and absence of inhibitions, it will not be difficult for husband and wife to sense each other's reactions. There are any number of ways in which the wife naturally shows her readiness for union, and the husband usually learns to interpret her physical and emotional responses. On the physical side, the wife's receptivity is evidenced by the appearance of a mucoid secretion around the vulva which comes from the glands of Bartholin, and it is usually well to wait until the external genitals become bathed with this moisture before actual entry takes place. The secretion moistens and lubricates the vulvar region and the opening to the vagina, making penetration easier and also heightening the sexual sensations. In the early days or even weeks of marriage physical tensions and emotional anxieties and restraints may inhibit the functioning of these glands, and the moisture may not readily appear. If this is so, it is advisable to use an artificial lubricant, in the form of a suitable type of aseptic greaseless jelly, which serves to make entry easier and more comfortable. This increases the likelihood of a mutually satisfactory climax, or orgasm.

The Orgasm of the Man

What exactly is the orgasm, Doctor?

Erotic stimulation produces a series of changes in almost every part of the body. When a man or woman becomes sexually aroused, the heart begins to beat faster, the blood pressure rises, and there is an increased flow of blood into the various organs, especially the genital organs—the penis, the clitoris, the inner labiae, the vaginal walls, the nipples of the breasts. At the same time there is a corresponding heightening of nervous tension which affects the entire body. As sexual stimulation proceeds, these changes become more and more marked until the moment of sudden release. This moment is the point commonly recognized as the orgasm. The term itself applies to the spasmodic contractions of the muscles surrounding the genitals, at the climax of the sex act. In the man the orgasm is accompanied by the ejaculation of the seminal fluid. The ampulla, the seminal vesicles and the prostate contract forcibly and expel their contents into the urethral canal, where the several secretions mix to form the seminal fluid. During the orgasm this fluid is ejaculated through the penis in a number of spurts by the rhythmic contractions of the surrounding musculature. The number and intensity of contractions experienced by the male vary in different individuals and also in the same person at different times, generally averaging from two or three to twenty, while the total quantity of the ejaculated seminal fluid amounts to nearly a teaspoonful.

The Orgasm of the Woman

Does the woman experience the same kind of reaction as the man at the time of the orgasm?

In the woman too the orgasm signifies the moment of the release of the accumulated tension. The descriptions which women give of their sensations during the orgasm vary considerably. "A feeling of completion," "a tingling all over," "waves coming one after another in ever-widening circles," "balloons bursting inside"—these are some of the phrases women have used to describe an orgasm. The actual physical manifestations consist in the main of throbbings, pulsations or contractions around the genital area and the lower abdomen.

These contractions are rhythmic and involuntary and are concentrated around the regions of the vulva, the vagina and the clitoris. Sometimes the contractions extend to other muscles of the body, too, and there may even be a few general convulsivelike movements at the time of orgasm. As a rule the local throbbings are fairly strong and distinct and the woman is usually definitely aware of their occurrence. Sometimes, however, the contractions are rather feeble and transient, so that the woman is barely conscious of them. The orgasm of the female subsides more gradually than that of the male, and its duration may therefore be more prolonged.

The emotional and erotic sensations as well as the behavior of the individual during the orgasm are subject to considerable variation in both the man and the woman, depending upon individual sensitivity and general intensity of emotional response. In some the sexual pleasure may be comparatively slight, while in others it may reach the height of mental and physical exultation. Between these two extremes there is a wide range of gradations of sensuous response. It is likely that these variations in the pattern of reaction may depend both upon basic constitutional differences and upon attitudes which, in part, have been inculcated in early life.

Is there a fluid discharged by the woman too at the time of her climax?

In the male, the ejaculation represents the discharge of his sperm into the genital tract of the woman and is therefore an essential part of the physiological process of reproduction. The woman, however, does not discharge her sex cells during intercourse, and there is, therefore, no emission on her part corresponding to the ejaculation of the male. The moisture of which she may be conscious during sexual excitement is due to the secretions of the glands of the vulva and is not a part of the orgasm. Some maintain that a certain amount of secretion is expelled from the uterus into the vagina during the climax, but further research has amply proved that this is not so.

Can either tell when the other has reached the climax?

The actual contractions of the sexual parts are not always felt by the mate, especially if the orgasms of the man and the woman are simultaneous. This is particularly true of the female contractions, which often cannot be felt at all by the male. However, the other manifestations which accompany the climax, the sudden release of the rising tension and the relaxation and sense of completion which follow, express themselves clearly in the behavior of the man and the woman and can generally be recognized by both.

If it takes the woman longer to reach a climax, is it difficult, then, for a couple to arrive at a mutually satisfactory sex relation?

There are great variations in women in the degree of sexual response and particularly in their ability to attain a satisfactory climax during intercourse. At the beginning of marriage, a woman's sexual desires may be still dormant, and there may, therefore, be little erotic response to the sexual act. Difficulty in achieving a mutual climax at this time should not be a source of anxiety. With a sympathetic understanding and with patience on the part of the husband, a harmonious adjustment may later be attained. If the woman is at all capable of reaching a climax, there should not be too much difficulty, even if her reaction time is slow. Delicacy in the sexual approach and stimulation, variety in the positions assumed during intercourse, and a general sensitivity and skill in the art of sexual love may, after a variable period of time, arouse the woman to a degree that will enable her to reach an orgasm with her husband. There are a number of women who may be unable to obtain complete sexual release even after a prolonged period of stimulation, but this is a problem which we shall discuss a little more fully at a later time.

Duration of the Sex Act

How long should sexual intercourse normally take?

That depends upon what the term includes. If we consider sexual intercourse to consist of the foreplay, the sexual union and also the afterplay—that is, the period of rest and relaxation which normally follows intercourse—the time would obviously be subject to any number of variations. Even if we consider coitus to extend only from intromission until the completion of the orgasm, there are also marked individual variations in its duration. The length of time that the man is able to retain an erection without an ejaculation, the ease or difficulty with which the woman is capable of reaching an orgasm, the degree of sexual tension at the time of intercourse, the frequency of the sexual relations, and many other elements determine the time factor on any occasion. While some men can prolong active coitus for fifteen or twenty minutes or more before ejaculation, others can hardly do so for more than a minute or so. Stekel states that few men are able to continue the sex act for more than five minutes, and Dickinson says that "the median man holds an erection from five to ten minutes."

From inquiries among a large number of couples it is my impression that these figures are rather high. There is a difference, of course, between simply "holding an erection," even in intromission, and maintaining it during active copulation. When both partners are passive, a man may learn to retain an erection for a comparatively long time, but with active coital movements the orgasm occurs, in most instances, in less than three minutes. From studies I have made, I should estimate the average duration of active coitus to be from one to two minutes. Similar figures, incidentally, were obtained by Kinsey in his findings on the sex behavior of American men. He too reports that the average duration of intercourse is about two minutes.

Coital Positions

You spoke before of a variety in the positions that may be assumed for intercourse. Does it make any difference which particular position is used, as far as sexual satisfaction is concerned?

Yes. Coital positions may affect the character and intensity of the sexual response. Ignorance concerning the positions suitable for the sex union is one of the frequent causes of awkwardness and difficulties in sexual adjustment, and this is therefore a question which deserves special consideration in any discussion of the art of marriage. We need not, of course, take up all the possible varieties of coital postures. Descriptions of a great many of them may be found in the erotic literature, but the majority are simply minor modifications of the usual positions. I shall consider only those which are most generally adopted and which appear to be most adequate and satisfactory from both a physical and a psychological standpoint.

Face-to-Face Position

The usual position for coitus and the one which is probably the most easily assumed is the anterior, front, or face-to-face posture. Here the woman lies on her back, with her thighs separated and her knees bent or drawn up toward her, while the man inclines over her, with the upper part of his body lightly in contact with hers. By supporting himself on his knees and on one or both hands or elbows, he avoids putting his weight upon the woman, thus making both more comfortable. Entrance can then be accomplished with ease, and there is close contact of the male and female organs. It is important to bear in mind, however, that in this position the knees of the woman would have to be bent and her thighs drawn up.

How far should the knees be drawn up?

The knees may be flexed only slightly, with the feet resting on the bed, or they may be drawn up so that the legs of the wife will encircle the husband's body. Some bending of the knees, however, is necessary. Many couples have difficulties in consummating the sexual union merely because they attempt to have intercourse with the wife lying straight on her back with her limbs outstretched or extended, a position which makes penetration very difficult. When the thighs and legs are straight, the inclination of the pelvis is such that the opening of the vagina points downward, and, as the male organ is elevated during erection, approximation is not easy. When the woman flexes her knees and separates her thighs, however, the entrance to the vagina is tilted upward, and at the same time it may be slightly opened, so that penetration can be accomplished with greater ease. In some instances it is even advisable to place a pillow underneath the wife's hips in order to increase further the tilt of the pelvis and bring the opening of the vagina forward. This permits deeper penetration and closer contact, and serves to heighten the sexual sensation and to facilitate the attainment of a climax.

After entry has been made, the wife may slowly straighten her knees and bring her thighs together. Although full penetration is not possible in this position, it affords closer approximation between the male organ and the external genitals of the woman, which is especially desirable when there is some difficulty with the potency of the man or the sexual response of the woman.

Side Position

A simple modification of the face-to-face posture is the side position. Here instead of lying on her back the woman lies on her side, with her knees drawn up and her thighs separated, while her husband lies facing her, resting between her limbs. If she lies on the right side, her right thigh is underneath him and her left is over his body. This posture is simple to adopt, and is comfortable because both the husband and the wife rest on the bed and very little weight is placed upon either.

There is another form of the side position, in which the couple also lie facing each other sideways. If the husband lies on his left side he draws up his left thigh, and the wife rests upon it. She then places her left leg over his body. This position sounds somewhat complicated, but it can be readily assumed, and many find it very comfortable. Ovid long ago advised the Roman ladies that "the simplest and the least fatiguing is to lie on your right side."

Reverse or Woman Superior Position

I understand that it is also possible to have intercourse with the woman in the upper position.

Yes. The woman may assume the superior, or upper, position and either sit astride or lie over her husband. The man lies flat on his back, with his thighs together, while the woman kneels or squats across him, and entrance is accomplished in this position. If the husband raises his knees slightly to support the wife's hips, she can bend her body forward over his, so that closer contact of the upper part of their bodies is possible, with full freedom for the touch and caress. In some instances a small pillow placed under the lower part of the husband's back makes this method more satisfactory and comfortable. In general, this position gives the woman greater freedom of motion, permits deeper and more complete penetration and closer sexual contact, and sometimes makes it easier for her to achieve a satisfactory climax.

Sitting Position

The sitting posture, in which the man sits on the edge of a chair or bed, and the woman sits, or, rather, is suspended, across his thighs, facing him, is also used occasionally. This is not especially practical or convenient, but in some instances it is found to be a stimulating variation.

Back Position

In the positions you have mentioned, the man and the woman always face each other during intercourse.

Yes, this is the characteristically human attitude in the sexual act at the present time. In their study *Patterns of Sexual Behavior,* Ford and Beach point out that all mammals except man copulate in a rear-entry, or back, position, with the male behind the female, but that in all known human societies rear entry is not the usual pattern of intercourse. It is, however, practiced occasionally in many areas of the world. In this position the woman lies on her side, with her back to her husband, and the man, lying on his side, approaches her from behind. She may also assume the so-called knee-chest position, kneeling face downward, with her elbows and chest resting on the bed, while the man kneels behind her. Aside from presenting an element of variety, and permitting closer compression of the urethral area and manual stimulation of the clitoris at the same time, there does not seem to be any particular advantage to this posture. It does not allow complete penetration; it often places a physical strain upon both the man and the woman; and, above all, it does not permit the face-to-face contact and caress which are so important an accompaniment of sexual intercourse among civilized peoples.

The Cross Position

Another position which has this drawback of not allowing face-to-face contact, but which nevertheless has certain advantages, is the cross, or scissors, position. The woman lies on her back, while the man lies on his side at right angles to her body and under her uplifted thighs, which rest on his hip. Among the advantages of this position are the ease with which it can be assumed and the fact that neither person bears any large part of the other's weight. The partners' legs can also be twined together in a variety of ways without making the motions of intercourse at all difficult. In this position manual contact with the vulva and the clitoris can easily be achieved by the male, and this is of importance where this type of stimulation is necessary to bring about a satisfactory response. As an alternative to the side or back position, the cross position is also useful during pregnancy, when no great weight should rest on the woman's abdomen.

I have mentioned the several positions which are probably the simplest and most convenient. There are a great many others indeed. Ovid, perhaps with true poetic license, said that "love has a thousand postures." To detail too large a number of them might only prove confusing and more of a hindrance than a help. As in other fields of sexual play, it is best, it seems to me, to allow for spontaneity and ingenuity on the part of the individual couple. After a while they will learn to adopt the postures which prove most comfortable and most satisfactory to them, and to vary the modes of coitus in accordance with changing needs and desires.

But aren't some of the positions you mentioned unnatural and abnormal?

I do not think that we can consider any particular method of sexual union as normal or abnormal. The use of one or another mode of intercourse is largely a matter of social, cultural and aesthetic traditions and attitudes. What is considered natural in one place may be regarded as quite the opposite in another. The inhabitants of Kamchatka use the side position for intercourse, supposedly because this is the mode of contact among fish, which constitute their chief food supply, and they regard anyone who practices coitus in any other fashion as committing a grave sin. In many primitive societies the general pattern of coitus is for the woman to lie on her back on the ground, with her legs spread and raised and her knees flexed, while the man squats or kneels in front of her. He then pulls her toward him, raising the lower part of her body so that her legs grasp him around his pelvic region. People using this method regard the European position as less effective and even as abnormal. Obviously, then, it is largely a question of environment, training and conventions as to whether a particular form of sex contact is considered normal or abnormal. One might say, indeed, that no position which is effective need be regarded as taboo or indecent, and that variety in the sexual approach is much to be desired for mutual sexual satisfaction.

The Epilogue to the Sex Act

Some time ago I saw a quotation to the effect that "all animals feel sad after intercourse." Is there any truth in this saying?

This statement, which was supposedly made by the Greek physician Galen many centuries ago, is still frequently quoted, yet I doubt whether there is really any psychological or physiological basis for it. The intense physical and mental excitement which usually precedes and accompanies the sex act may be followed by a period of some languor and at times even of fatigue or exhaustion, but this does not imply sadness or mental depression. On the contrary, a satisfactory sexual experience is more apt to leave the individual with a sense of well-being and agreeable repose.

As a rule the sexual embrace should be followed by an afterglow, a feeling of gratification and relaxation. This period is really a part of the sex union and is important to the completion of the act. When a couple are physically, emotionally and sexually well attuned, the sexual embrace should be succeeded by a sense of closeness and intimacy.

We have spoken at some length today about the technique of the sexual relation, and we shall discuss many other related problems next time. I should like, however, to stress again at this point that the art of sex is but one phase, although an important one, of the art of marriage. Marriage is a complex relationship and, to be satisfactory, requires any number of personality adjustments and adaptations. Happiness in marriage does not come spontaneously. It is not a gift which is bestowed, but a goal to be attained. Anything, therefore, that contributes to the art of marriage deserves understanding and consideration.

In the books I have already suggested are many chapters dealing with the subjects we have discussed today. I shall mention several others in which you may find much instructive information.

Bibliography

Brecher, Ruth and Edward, eds., *An Analysis of Human Sexual Response.* Signet Books, New American Library, 1966.

Brown, Fred, and Kempton, Rudolph T., *Sex Questions and Answers: A Guide to Happy Marriage.* McGraw-Hill paperback, 1960.

Butterfield, Oliver M., *Sex Life in Marriage.* Emerson, 1962.

——, *Sexual Harmony in Marriage.* Emerson, 1967. Also in paperback.

Davis, Maxine, *Sexual Responsibility in Marriage.* Dial Press, 1963.

Ellis, Havelock, *The Psychology of Sex.* Emerson, 1938. Also in New American Library paperback.

Exner, Max J., M.D., *The Sexual Side of Marriage.* Norton, 1932.

Ford, Clellan S., and Beach, Frank A., *Patterns of Sexual Behavior.* Harper, 1951.

Gottlieb, Bernard S. and Sophie B., *What You Should Know About Marriage.* Bobbs-Merrill, 1962.

Kinsey, Alfred C., Pomeroy, W. B., and Martin, Clyde E., *Sexual Behavior in the Human Male.* Saunders, 1948.

Kinsey, Alfred C., and others, *Sexual Behavior in the Human Female.* Saunders, 1953. Also in Pocket Books paperback.

Masters, W. H., and Johnson, V. E., *Human Sexual Response.* Little, Brown, 1966.

Naismith, Grace, *Private and Personal.* McKay, 1966.

Rainer, Jerome and Julia, *Sexual Pleasure in Marriage.* Simon and Schuster, 1959.

Robie, W. F., M.D., *The Art of Love.* Brown, 1962. Also in Parliament paperback.

Van de Velde, T. H., M.D., *Ideal Marriage,* rev. ed. Random House, 1965.

CHAPTER VIII

SEXUAL ADJUSTMENTS AND MALADJUSTMENTS

Last time we spoke of the nature and technique of the sexual union and of the importance of attaining a mutually satisfactory sex relationship; today I should like to discuss with you certain types of sexual disharmonies which sometimes seriously affect an otherwise successful marriage. Young people about to marry should be aware of these potential difficulties and not find themselves totally bewildered and distressed when an unexpected problem does arise. They should know something of what Balzac calls the "sandbanks, the reefs, the rocks, the breakers, the currents" on the sea of matrimony, so that they may be able to steer their barks clear of the dangerous areas. Much unhappiness in marriage can be prevented by a more realistic understanding of the potential difficulties which may be encountered.

Sex and Marital Harmony

Would you say that most of the troubles in marriage are the result of sex maladjustments?

No, of course not. Any number of factors play a part in the adjustment of two people in marriage—their personalities, the degree of their emotional security, their mutual compatibility, their social and economic situation, family relationships, and many others. I intend to discuss some of these with you in greater detail later on. The sex factor is, however, of major importance in marriage, and directly and indirectly it also influences many other aspects of the relationship between husband and wife. If sexual disharmonies can, therefore, be prevented or corrected, a successful marriage can be more readily achieved.

I want to stress, however, the fact that, while unsatisfactory sex relations can lead to other serious dissatisfactions in marriage, maladjustment in other areas can, on the other hand, affect the sexual harmony of a couple. A husband and wife who are congenial and happy in their personal relations may readily overlook certain disharmonies in their sexual life, while the same sexual disharmonies are apt to be magnified into serious proportions by a couple who are not compatible and who have frequent marital conflicts on other grounds.

Would you say, Doctor, that more sexual maladjustments are encountered in marriage today than formerly?

Perhaps so, but it is also likely that we have now become more fully aware of sexual problems and that they are therefore more frequently brought to our attention. For one thing, the economic and cultural emancipation of woman has freed her from many of the inhibitions of the past and has made her more fully conscious of her own sexual needs. When the wife accepted sexual relations merely as a duty, her husband's and her own sexual capacities and reactions did not often come into question. Today women are beginning to realize more fully the importance of a mutually satisfying sex relation and are therefore becoming more aware of any deficiencies or disharmonies that may exist.

Another probable cause for the increase in sexual disabilities are the tensions, insecurities and emotional conflicts in modern life. Human sex behavior is determined by two factors—instinctive drives and social influences. In our society the group assumes a dominant control over sex conduct, and there is therefore frequently an emotional conflict between desire and inhibitions. Among primitive people, where social life and sexual standards are more simple and natural, sexual inadequacies are not often encountered. In our culture, however, the many tensions of daily living have a disturbing effect on sexual function and capacity, and these tensions may lead to many disharmonies in the sex life of a couple.

Difficulties in Consummation of Sexual Union

Are sexual difficulties likely to occur at the very beginning of marriage?

Yes, they may develop from the start and are apt to make the first weeks or months of marriage very trying. Difficulties, for instance, may be encountered even in the consummation of the sexual union. "Consummation" is the legal term for the penetration of the vagina by the penis. Newly married couples are at times unsuccessful in completing the sex union, and they may be very much astonished and disconcerted by such an unexpected complication. These difficulties may persist for weeks or months and prove very disturbing to both husband and wife.

Ignorance of Sex Technique

But why should a couple be unable to consummate their marriage?

Several causes may account for it. Ignorance of the mechanism of coitus and consequent awkwardness in technique, an involuntary contraction of the muscles around the entrance to the vagina which makes penetration impossible, persistent pain to the woman during attempts at intercourse, anatomical abnormalities, lack of sufficient potency on the part of the husband—these are some of the causes of the failure to achieve a satisfactory physical union.

Let me cite to you, as an example, a case where the failure of consummation was due entirely to ignorance of technique. This couple had been married for eleven months. They were very much in love and their marriage was generally very satisfactory, except that their attempts at coitus were unsuccessful and incomplete. This situation was now causing a serious rift in their relations, and they decided to seek medical advice. An examination disclosed that entry had not yet taken place and that the wife was still a virgin. The difficulty was found to be due simply to a lack of understanding of the mechanics of intercourse. Neither of them had any knowledge, for example, of the positions to be assumed during the sex relation. When they attempted coitus, the wife would remain rigid and tense and lie with her thighs and legs fully extended, a position in which entry is hardly possible. She had no idea that it was necessary to bend or draw up and separate her knees. An explanation of the cause of their difficulties, and some instruction in sex anatomy and technique, helped solve their problem in a short time.

I can understand the wife's lack of knowledge, but it seems rather surprising that the husband should have been equally ignorant.

In this particular instance the husband had had no sexual experiences prior to marriage. However, even when a man has had premarital relations, it does not necessarily mean that he acquires sufficient sexual knowledge. Premarital experiences are sometimes limited to women who take the initiative themselves and guide the man in the sex act. After marriage, however, it is the man who has to play the role of initiator, and he may then find himself quite unequipped for the purpose.

Vaginismus and Genital Spasm

Is it only a question, then, of lack of knowledge?

No, not all of the early difficulties are due to ignorance or lack of skill in the art of love. Sometimes it is the woman's reactions and attitudes which make intercourse difficult. Many women, as I mentioned last time, have a tendency to resist sex relations at first. Ordinarily this resistance soon disappears and normal coitus is established. In some cases, however, it persists for weeks, months and even years, and constitutes a serious obstacle to a satisfactory sexual adjustment. Here, for instance, is a typical history of such a case. This couple had been married for a year and a half, but the marriage had not yet been consummated, and the wife still had an intact hymen. The husband had normal sexual desires and potency, yet penetration seemed impossible. Whenever intercourse was attempted, the wife would become frightened and tense, would resist his approach and draw back in a defensive attitude. Both had been looking forward eagerly to a perfectly happy union, and they were greatly bewildered by the unexpected difficulties they were meeting. By now they were certain that there was some physical abnormality which made sex relations impossible, and that they were sexually mismated and hopelessly incompatible. An examination showed that the wife was physically normal, and that the failure of penetration was due to a muscular spasm, a forcible and involuntary contraction of the muscles around the entrance to the vagina, which made intromission impossible. Such a spasm, sometimes called vaginismus, is not infrequently the cause of sexual difficulties early in marriage.

In such cases, Doctor, does the woman consciously resist because she objects to the relation?

No, the resistance is in the nature of a reflex action which is beyond her voluntary control. The woman may be entirely normal in every other respect, she may even have strong sexual desires and be both willing and eager to submit to the sexual embrace, yet every time intercourse is attempted a reflex spasm of the genital muscles occurs which definitely prevents entry. Neither reasoning nor persuasion will have any effect. Forcible attempts merely lead to greater fear and serve to aggravate the situation. We have called this condition "genital spasm."

Causes of Genital Spasm

What causes this spasm? Is it due to nervousness?

This type of involuntary tightening of the muscles surrounding the lower part of the vagina may be due to either physical or emotional factors. Any local genital condition, for instance, which makes intercourse painful is apt to result in a muscular spasm. In most instances, however, the genital spasm represents an unconscious defense mechanism against sexual relations. Fears and anxieties, sexual inhibitions and taboos inculcated in early life, an upsetting sexual experience in youth—any of these may be responsible for the development of this type of muscular spasm at marriage.

How can early experiences or impressions cause this resistance to develop later on?

Well, because of the furtiveness with which sexual topics are generally treated by parents, the sex relation may become associated in the mind of the child with a feeling of sin, shame and guilt. A girl, furthermore, is often taught from infancy to avoid touching her genitals lest some serious harm befall her. As a result she is likely to develop the feeling that she must always be on guard against any injury to the genital area. Even though in later life the young woman may become emancipated from the sex taboos, she may still retain many of the inhibitions and protective attitudes of her childhood, and these may seriously interfere with her reactions and responses after marriage. She may involuntarily shrink from intercourse and set up a defensive mechanism in the form of this genital spasm. The outer resistance is but an expression of an unconscious inner resistance to sexual union.

Are such inhibitions really carried over into marriage? I should think that in the intimate daily life of two people feelings of this kind would soon disappear.

It is quite true that after marriage the early tensions and resistances often disappear and normal sex relations are established. Sometimes, however, they do persist for a long time, particularly when the husband is unskilled and awkward in his approach. It is not easy for a woman to throw off at once the inhibitions and taboos she had accumulated during a lifetime, simply because the marriage ceremony has given her a legal and social sanction for sex relations. If the husband is impatient and unsympathetic in his attitude and behavior he may only aggravate her anxieties and increase her resistance.

How can such fears be removed, then?

The best way, of course, is to prevent their occurrence. This implies an intelligent sex education in youth. The attitudes implanted in the mind of a girl early in life may profoundly influence her sex behavior in later years. Directly and indirectly parents impose their own values and their own standards upon their children. A sense of what parents assume to be right or wrong, proper or improper, good or bad, is generally transmitted to the children in the course of daily life. Parents should, therefore, be aware of the lasting influence they sometimes have in molding and conditioning the sex pattern of their children.

Furthermore, attention should be given to educating and preparing young people for the marital relation. The husband, especially, should learn to realize that he has to exercise patience and restraint at the beginning, and that he must make every effort to win the complete confidence and trust of his wife. Let me read to you some advice on this subject from Vatsyayana's *Kama Sutra*, written over sixteen hundred years ago:

Women, being of a tender nature, want tender beginnings, and when they are forcibly approached by men with whom they are but slightly acquainted, they sometimes suddenly become haters of sexual connection, and sometimes even haters of the male sex. The man should, therefore, approach his bride according to her liking, and should make use of those devices by which he may be able to establish himself more and more into her confidence.

This recommendation made so long ago is still applicable today and offers excellent advice for the prevention of many sexual disharmonies.

Treatment of Genital Spasm

But if this tension or spasm does develop after marriage, what should be done about it?

It is essential, first, for both husband and wife to understand the origin and significance of this condition. Once the nature of the difficulty is recognized, the chances of correcting it are so much greater. Instruction or reinstruction in the physiology, psychology and art of the sexual relation, a reorientation of the wife's attitude, the correction of any physical abnormality, and, when necessary, an artificial dilatation of the hymen are usually sufficient to remedy the condition.

Painful Coitus

You mentioned that pain during intercourse may be a cause of sexual difficulties. Did you mean the pain caused by the breaking of the hymen?

No, the pain caused by stretching of the hymen is only temporary, and by the end of a week or so coitus should not be accompanied by any discomfort. The painful disturbance I spoke of results from other factors. Physical anomalies, inflammations of the external or internal sex organs, irritations due to clumsy and awkward attempts at coitus—these and other conditions may be responsible for pain during sexual union. If the discomfort is severe enough, it may render sexual intercourse so unpleasant for the wife that she may even try to avoid it altogether.

Here, for example, is the story of a woman who began to be troubled with pain during intercourse soon after marriage. The pain persisted long after the hymen was fully dilated, and it became more acute as time went on. After a while it reached a stage where sex relations became so unpleasant to her and so unsatisfactory to her husband that for many months they practically avoided all sexual contact. They ascribed their difficulties to a sexual incompatibility or to a disproportion of their sex organs, and they each secretly regarded the marriage as a failure. An examination of the wife disclosed the presence of an inflammation of the vulva and the vagina, which responded readily to local treatment. The relief of the condition soon led to the disappearance of the pain during intercourse, and eventually entirely normal and satisfactory sex relations were established. I am citing the case because the history is rather characteristic of this type of sexual disturbance. Painful intercourse is not at all infrequent and may become a source of serious marital dissatisfaction and unhappiness. It is important not to let it continue too long without medical attention, for simple medical care and advice may often relieve the difficulty.

Sexual Frigidity in Women

Aren't there many women, though, who avoid sex relations mainly because they have little sex desire?

Well, there are wide variations in the intensity of the sex urge in both men and women. Some people are "highly sexed," with a strong sexual drive, while others have comparatively little or no sex desire. Between these two extremes there are many gradations.

Sexual coldness, or frigidity, as it is called, is rather frequent among women and may manifest itself in a variety of ways. Some women lack any sex urge and have, so to speak, no sexual appetite; others have fairly strong desires and can become easily aroused, but they experience little or no pleasure from the sex act itself; and there are women who even have a positive distaste for, or aversion to, intercourse, and who regard the sexual relation merely as an unpleasant marital duty.

When a woman is frigid, does it mean that she has no sexual feelings at all or merely that she does not respond to a particular mate?

This is a point which has to be determined in each instance. A woman may be totally frigid and have no sexual desire under any circumstances, or her sexual coolness may be only temporary and relative in degree, the result of a number of marital factors. Absolute and permanent frigidity is rare. "Frigidity," says Dickinson, "is not a fixed state which comes on whole and is borne to the grave." The woman who has no sexual feeling may be merely one who has not yet discovered the form of erotic stimulation which would bring a response in her case. In our experience, we have found that most women who claim complete sexual indifference give a history of some degree of sexual arousal at one time or another and of sexual gratification from masturbation or some other form of sex play. In these cases it is not a question of the total absence of any sex urge, but, rather, of the suppression of erotic feelings, or of failure to respond to a particular form of sexual approach or stimulation.

Total frigidity, then, is probably very rare. Very few women are altogether cold and unresponsive. On the other hand, a relative degree of sexual coolness and lack of response exists among a fairly high percentage of women. In reply to a questionnaire sent by Katherine Davis to one thousand married women, only sixty-two per cent of the wives stated that sex relations were definitely pleasurable to them. Sixteen per cent claimed that they were "neutral" toward sexual union, ten per cent said that the act was definitely distasteful to them, and the remaining twelve per cent were doubtful concerning their reactions. In other words, at least twenty-six per cent of the women could be considered sexually unresponsive. A similar incidence of deficiency in sexual response was found among the patients of the Margaret Sanger Research Bureau. We have been recording the patients' attitudes toward sex relations as a part of the Bureau's clinical histories, and in an analysis of some nine thousand of these records it was found that seventy-six per cent of the women reported what may be considered a normal sexual attitude, twenty per cent stated that they were indifferent to the sexual act, and four per cent claimed a definite aversion to intercourse. Here too, then, we find that about one out of every four women was sexually unresponsive.

Causes of Female Frigidity

What accounts for this lack of sexual desire? Is it due to any physical abnormality?

The normal development and expression of the sexual impulse is dependent upon both physiological and psychological factors, and consequently either physical or emotional disturbances may affect the extent or intensity of sex desire. Physiologically, there is considerable evidence that in animals, at least, sexual activity is controlled mainly by hormones. In female animals, for instance, the periods of increased sexual desire are closely associated with the processes of ovulation and with the increased hormone production which occurs at this time. If the ovaries are removed, then the artificial administration of the female sex hormone stimulates the sexual activity of the animal. While in women the sexual drive is dependent to a much lesser degree upon hormone production, disturbances in the functions of the internal glands may also lead to a diminution or loss of sex desire.

However, the available data indicate that in human beings social, cultural and emotional factors play a more significant part in the development of the sexual impulse. As we go up the scale of animal evolution, sexual activity and receptivity become less and less dependent upon hormones and progressively more upon the nervous system and the brain. Sex behavior becomes less of an instinctive and more of a learned process. Outside factors play an increasingly important role in influencing sex activity and behavior. A decrease in sex desire may therefore be caused not by any physical or physiological deficiency, but by environmental influences. For example, Kinsey found that the marked variations in the degree of sexual response of women depended to a considerable degree upon differences in their social and educational levels.

Well, then, Doctor, if a woman finds herself frigid in her marital relations, does the cause lie with her or with the particular marriage?

In a large percentage of cases the lack of response is undoubtedly due to influences which existed long before the marriage, some of which can be traced back to childhood. A woman may be frigid because she was brought up in a subzero atmosphere. The high incidence of frigidity among women is largely the result of faulty sex education and an inability to become freed from fears and inhibitions acquired in early life. I have already mentioned some of the factors which can disturb the sex response in women, and these conditions may, under certain circumstances, completely inhibit any sex desire.

Among the chief causes of frigidity are fear and anxiety, fear of sex, fear of surrender, fear of pain, fear of bodily harm, fear of pregnancy, and fear of disapproval. Many of these fears develop during childhood and adolescence. If, for instance, a girl is brought up with the idea that the sexual relation is animallike, degrading and immoral, if she is constantly warned against any physical expression of love, she may grow up with the strong feeling that sex is inherently vulgar, shameful or sinful, and this attitude may not readily change after the wedding. She may become emancipated intellectually and yet remain emotionally enslaved by her childhood fears and inhibitions.

Let me read to you, as an illustration, a paragraph from a letter which bears upon this point. This letter came from a young married woman, a college graduate, deeply attached to her husband, physically normal, but troubled because of her lack of sex desire. In telling of her early life she writes:

I always considered sexual intercourse a sign of extreme weakness, sinful, and not to be condoned. Up to about sixteen years of age I had the notion that a woman was destined to have a certain number of children, and that only one sexual congress of the parents was necessary. That was the only way I could explain why my parents, who were extremely poor, should keep on having babies. Because of the extreme poverty in our home and the frequent additions to the family, I worked up a strong dread of marriage and of the sexual act. . . . My dread of intercourse and what I considered the misery of married life even increased as I grew older.

Here we find a number of factors—the total lack of an intelligent sex education, the association of intercourse with weakness and sin, the dread of childbearing—all of which had obviously combined to inhibit any normal sex expression by this young woman. As a matter of fact, it took some time before she was finally able to overcome these early impressions and repressions.

But what about the marriage itself? Isn't the husband sometimes responsible for lack of desire on the part of his wife?

Yes, that's quite true. The lack of desire may be due to factors which exist in the particular mating. The sexual responses of the woman are usually closely bound up with her emotional reactions and with her attitude toward her mate. A man can ordinarily obtain sexual satisfaction even with a woman for whom he has little or no feeling. A woman, however, is not likely to respond to a man for whom she has no affection, or who does not express tenderness or consideration for her. A wife's sexual reaction to her husband may thus depend more upon the everyday expressions of his feeling for her—his attitude, his manner, his interest in her as an individual. If he shows no consideration for her as a person, she may eventually lose any interest in him as a sexual partner.

Furthermore, in cases of frigidity, the husband's sexual capacity and behavior must also be taken into consideration. "It takes two persons to make one frigid woman," says Dickinson. If the husband is awkward and clumsy in his approach, if he lacks any art or skill in sexual love, if he is inept in his attempts to arouse and stimulate his wife, she may never be fully awakened sexually and may remain quite unresponseive to sexual contact. Then again, if the husband's sexual capacity is inadequate, if he has a low degree of sexual desire, if his ejaculations come on rapidly or prematurely, or if he practices coitus interruptus and withdraws before the wife is sufficiently aroused, the wife may develop an antipathy and even a definite aversion to sexual union. Either she may not become stimulated at all or else the repeated frustrations will gradually lead to a loss of any pleasurable sensation and eventually to a loss on her part of desire for sexual intimacy. If time after time she is left in "mid-air," she may after a while refuse to leave the ground altogether.

The Treatment of Frigidity

Suppose a man finds after marriage that his wife is unresponsive, is there anything he can do about it?

First of all, one has to realize that the sexual impulse of the woman may normally remain dormant for a long period. It may not, in fact, develop to its full capacity until she is well beyond her twenties, or even later. Moll once divided the sexual urge into two elements: the impulse toward general bodily contact, "to approach, touch, and kiss a person of the opposite sex," and the impulse toward sex union, toward the relief of sexual tension. In the girl the desire for bodily contact is at first, at least, much more strongly developed than the desire for genital contact, and the caress, the embrace and the kiss may be more gratifying to her than actual sex union. Some women have strong sex desires from the very beginning of marriage, but often enough it takes months or even years before the sexual feelings of the wife are sufficiently awakened so that she consciously and actively desires full sexual contact and takes pleasure in the sex act. The lack of complete response at first may therefore be only due to the fact that the latent sexual capacities of the wife have not yet been fully developed.

If the frigidity persists, however, the measures which may have to be taken to overcome or correct the condition will depend upon the nature and the cause in the individual instance. Adequate sexual education or, more usually, re-education, of the wife and of the husband, with a reorientation of the wife's attitudes to allay baseless apprehensions and fears, instruction in the technique and art of love, the provision of satisfactory and reliable methods for the prevention of conception—these and other medical and psychotherapeutic measures are often of great value.

It is especially important that the husband acquire the knowledge and understanding, the delicacy and the skill, the ability and the art of arousing the sexual impulses of his wife and of finding the means of gratification which are most satisfactory in her individual case.

As far as the wife is concerned, she must make every effort to obtain an insight into the nature of her disability, to recognize her deficiency, and to appreciate the importance of correcting it. Every now and then a woman will state with a considerable show of satisfaction and pride that she is indifferent to sexual contact and that she derives no pleasure from sex union. She looks upon her sexual anesthesia as an indication of her moral virtue and spiritual superiority. "Oh," she will say, "I'm not that kind, sex doesn't mean anything to me. I wouldn't care if he never touched me." Obviously such an attitude is in itself a contributing cause of her sexual failure. The woman should be made to understand that a mutual sexual response is of paramount importance to marital harmony, and that her frigidity is not a matter for pride and satisfaction, but a sign of a physical or emotional inadequacy. She must realize that her husband cannot long retain his sexual ardor if she herself is totally unresponsive, and that for her own welfare, as well as for the happiness of the marriage, she should endeavor to develop a sexual interest and response.

As a matter of fact, I should go a step further and suggest that even if her sexual desire is not very strong a wife need not constantly emphasize the fact of her indifference to her husband, or always inform him of her lack of response. At times it may even be well for her to simulate an interest in the sex act, for this in itself may help to create a greater marital harmony and aid in gradually correcting her sexual indifference.

Orgasm Incapacity

Last time you mentioned that some women have difficulty in reaching a satisfactory climax during intercourse. Is this condition a form of frigidity?

The inability to attain an orgasm is really quite distinct from frigidity. In frigidity, either the woman experiences no sexual desire at all or else the sex act gives rise to no pleasurable sensations; in orgasm incapacity, the desire may be quite normal and the sensations during the act even intense, but the final climax is not reached.

This failure to reach an orgasm is, in fact, another frequent source of sexual disharmony. Ordinarily the completion of the sex act is characterized by a rather distinct emotional and physical reaction, by keen erotic sensations and by the local muscular contractions which constitute the orgasm. Many women, however, rarely or even never reach this culminating reaction, and this inadequacy sometimes leads to marital unhappiness and discord.

Is difficulty in reaching an orgasm a common occurrence?

Yes, orgasm incapacity is more frequent than is generally recognized. It is perhaps the most usual sexual complaint of women who are otherwise entirely normal. The capacity to reach a climax cannot, however, be definitely classified as either positive or negative. It may vary in degree and intensity from a very transient sensation to a very profound physical experience. Some women reach a satisfactory climax during every sexual relation, others only once in a while, as once in every three, four or more cohabitations; some women experience an orgasm very rarely, only when a special combination of physiological and emotional circumstances makes a complete sexual release possible, and others never reach this culmination, although they may derive a considerable degree of satisfaction from the sex relation.

As far as the frequency of these variations is concerned, the figures of several studies on this subject may be illuminating. In his detailed analysis of one hundred couples, Hamilton found that forty-six of the hundred wives had what he termed "a very inferior or wholly lacking orgasm capacity." Dickinson, in a study of 310 cases, found that out of every five women two reached an orgasm fairly frequently, one attained it "sometimes," and two did not reach any climax. In the series from the Margaret Sanger Research Bureau, out of over eighty-five hundred women thirty-four per cent reported that they had experienced an orgasm "usually," forty-six per cent experienced it occasionally or "rarely," and twenty per cent stated that they had never reached an orgasm. The orgasm capacity of another group of three thousand women whose records we have analyzed showed somewhat similar figures. Some forty-one per cent reached an orgasm regularly, forty-three per cent experienced it only occasionally or rarely, and sixteen per cent never attained the final reaction. As the women in these several studies did not come to us primarily because of any sexual difficulties or maladjustment, the figures can be considered as a fair index of the average status of women as far as orgasm experience is concerned.

Why is it that so many women have difficulty in reaching a climax during intercourse?

There is no general agreement yet as to the actual cause of orgasm failure in so high a percentage of normal women. Some, indeed, maintain that the orgasm of the female is not a universal physiological phenomenon, and that the female animal generally does not reach any particular climax during sexual mating. They regard the development of the orgasm reflex in women as a special human attribute, an attribute which is still not deeply rooted in her organism and is therefore subject to frequent and wide variations and anomalies.

Causes of Orgasm Incapacity

It seems to me, however, that the failure of response must be looked for in some more specific causes, either physical or emotional in character. From the physical side the orgasm difficulty may in part, at least, be accounted for by the relative positions of the erogenous zones of the woman's genital organs. There is one point which is of particular significance in this respect. As we have already noted, a woman's erotic sensations are much more diffuse than a man's, though they are also centered in and around the clitoris. Before sexual relations are established, erotic gratification is often obtained through stimulation of the external genitals and sometimes of the clitoris. Repeated excitation of this area during youth and adolescence, either from self-stimulation or from sex play, may further concentrate the sensuous feelings in this region. Later, when sex relations are begun, erotic response is expected to be achieved through more intimate contact with the vaginal walls, but in many women the vagina is apparently not erotically sensitive. This is why so many women will reach an orgasm with comparative ease upon stimulation of the external genitals, yet they will not reach a climax from vaginal contact and may even have very little or no sexual gratification from the act of intercourse.

But why is it that the vagina itself is not highly sensitive?

Well, perhaps because the clitoris and the inner labiae of the human female are much more richly supplied with sensory nerve endings than are the walls of the vagina. The woman's erotic sensations during intercourse come largely from stimulation of the areas around the entrance to the vagina, rather than from internal vaginal contact.

Isn't the clitoris stimulated during intercourse?

Apparently not directly or not sufficiently. This, it seems to me, is one of the anomalies in the sexual physiology of the human female. If you look at the diagram of the female genitals you will notice that the clitoris is situated about an inch or more above the orifice of the vagina. During intercourse there is, therefore, comparatively little direct contact between the male organ and the clitoris. It is only when penetration is deep and complete that there may be external pressure upon the clitoris and the surrounding area. The difficulties in sexual response which many young women experience at the beginning of their marital relations may sometimes be due to the fact that penetration is not complete at this time and hence the contact of the organs is not sufficiently close.

However, in responsive women with a good attitude toward sex, and with adequate foreplay, orgasm may be reached in any coital position, even though the clitoris and clitoridial area are not subjected to direct pressure or stimulation. The importance of the clitoris in the individual case can be judged only when considered in connection with the other physical and emotional problems which enter into the sexual relationship.

Then emotional factors can also influence a woman's ability to have an orgasm, Doctor?

To discuss the various psychic or emotional conditions which may be responsible for orgasm difficulties in the female, I should have to repeat much of what I have already said in connection with the other forms of sexual disharmonies. The same psychological factors which may lead to genital spasm or to frigidity may also result in orgasm incapacity. Faulty sex instruction, inhibitions and repressions, fears and anxieties, sexual shocks of one kind or another, infantile fixations, homosexual or other forms of sexual deviation— any of these may lead to difficulties in orgasm response. The inability to reach a climax may represent an unconscious reluctance to surrender completely to the sexual embrace.

Is it possible to tell from a medical examination whether or not a woman will be able to reach a climax during intercourse?

A woman's capacity for sexual response cannot be determined

from a physical examination. The size and thickness of the clitoris, or of its hood, or of the labiae, may give some indication of the capacity for sexual arousal, but there are no physical signs which will show whether a woman will or will not be able to reach an orgasm during intercourse. The inability of a woman to react fully to the sexual relation is rarely related to any specific organic abnormality.

Does the husband's sexual capacity or technique influence the wife's ability to reach a climax?

Yes, in many instances a wife's failure to reach a satisfactory climax may be due to her husband's sexual inadequacy. A woman's sexual-reaction time is as a rule much lower than that of the man; it usually takes her longer both to become erotically aroused and to attain an orgasm. If the husband looks upon the sexual relation merely as a means of satisfying his own biological urge, if he makes no effort to arouse his wife's desires before sexual union, or if he can maintain an erection for only a brief period and reaches his orgasm quickly, the wife may not be stimulated to a degree that enables her also to reach a climax before the completion of the act. This is one reason, perhaps, why a woman will sometimes respond fully with one man and yet fail to do so with another.

I should emphasize, however, that the extent of the woman's orgasm response is not a problem only of the husband's sexual vigor or skill. We constantly come across cases in which the husband's potency is far above the average and his sexual approach entirely adequate, yet even after a long period of precoital play and a considerable prolongation of the sexual act his wife may not be able to achieve an orgasm. Here some of the other physical or emotional factors which I have mentioned may be responsible for the condition.

If a woman is frigid or is unable to reach an orgasm, would it in any way indicate that she has little feeling for her husband or that she is not sufficiently attracted to him physically?

Many men believe that the failure of a woman to respond fully during intercourse is a sign of her lack of affection or devotion. As a matter of fact, an inability to attain an orgasm does not at all indicate a lack of love or attraction. A woman may be profoundly and sincerely attached to a man and yet be unable to obtain any keen satisfaction from sexual relations with him. A large number of women, as we have already noted, obtain greater pleasure from intimate love play than they do from actual intercourse, and the failure to reach an orgasm during sexual union is therefore not a sign of insufficient physical or emotional attraction.

Effect of Orgasm Incapacity

Is the failure to reach a satisfactory orgasm apt to affect a woman's health in any way?

First, I should like to stress the fact that even if a woman does not attain an intense climax she may still derive a great deal of satisfaction from the sex act. Some women, indeed, are not aware of any orgasm problem until they learn about it from a conversation or a book. Only then do they become concerned about their lack of complete gratification from their sex experiences. As a matter of fact, some of the literary descriptions of the manifestations of the orgasm are more ideal than real, and they often lead men and women to expect sensations which are but rarely experienced. When D. H. Lawrence, for instance, in speaking of a woman at the completion of the sex act, says that she experienced "pure deepening whirlpools of sensation, swirling deeper and deeper through all her tissues and consciousness till she was one perfect concentric fluid of feeling, and she lay there crying in unconscious inarticulate cries," he may give a very lyrical description of an intense climactic reaction, but it does not represent the sensations of the average woman. Yet I have known women who, having read this or similar passages, were greatly disturbed because they were not reaching such ecstatic reactions, and men who were much perturbed because their wives did not show such an intensity of feeling, although in reality their mutual response was quite satisfactory.

If an actual orgasm deficiency does exist, its effect upon the woman would depend largely upon the intensity of her sexual desires and the degree of her excitation at the time of the relation. If her sexual impulse is not very strong, or if she is aroused only to a slight degree, the absence of the orgasm will hardly have any harmful effects.

On the other hand, if she has been very much stimulated, the failure to reach a climax may leave her in a state of frustration which may prove physiologically and emotionally disturbing. During erotic excitation there is a marked local congestion of the sexual organs, as well as a general physical and emotional tension. With the completion of the act, if a climax is reached, there is a gradual release, or detumescence, followed by a sense of fulfillment and relaxation. In the absence of an orgasm, however, the relief is not complete, and the woman may remain for some time in an unsatisfied and restless condition. Repeated experiences of this kind may eventually lead to various physical or emotional disturbances.

Orgasm and Fertility

Would the failure to reach a climax have any bearing upon a woman's ability to conceive?

There is little relation, as far as we know, between orgasm capacity and fertility, and, indeed, the orgasm is not a biological necessity for the female. The male climax is, of course, essential for reproduction; it is during the climax that the seminal fluid is ejaculated into the female genital tract, and without an ejaculation insemination could not take place. In the woman, the orgasm plays no such physiological role. The female does not discharge any specific fluid during the climax, and the release of the egg from the ovary, in the human species, is not dependent upon the orgasm. Some have maintained that the orgasm aids impregnation because during the culmination of the sex act the uterus presumably contracts and expands, producing a suctionlike effect which draws in the seminal fluid, but this point has been amply proved to be only a fantasy. At any rate it is quite certain that women can and do become pregnant without reaching an orgasm. We have records of a large number of women who were fertile and bore many children without ever having attained an orgasm during all the years of their marriage. The failure to reach a climax, then, does not materially affect the woman's capacity to conceive.

The Treatment of Orgasm Incapacity

What can be done to overcome a woman's inability to reach a climax?

The means which may have to be employed to correct an incapacity to reach orgasm will depend largely upon the nature and cause of the deficiency. If the husband's sexual technique or capacity is at fault, this must obviously be corrected. If it is a question of the wife's attitude toward sex, it may be necessary to relieve some of her inhibitions and her conscious and unconscious fears. In some instances, therapy may be advisable. A warm, understanding and patient attitude on the part of the physician is very important, but the physician's ingenuity will often be greatly taxed in the management of this condition.

As far as the husband's sexual approach is concerned, I have already spoken at some length concerning the precoital play and the necessity of arousing and stimulating his wife before sexual union. The husband should not enter the vagina until the wife is sufficiently aroused, and he should try as far as he can to prolong the sex act so that she may have the opportunity to respond more fully.

Occasionally a change in the coital position is helpful. There are women who, perhaps because of the anatomical relations of their genital organs, are able to reach a climax satisfactorily in a particular posture, as, for instance, in the reverse or in the back position, but not in the usual one, and it is advisable to make use of the position most adequate for the couple. The husband and wife should feel free to discuss the problem between themselves and to indicate to each other the types of sex play which are most stimulating and gratifying to each of them. They should experiment and vary their sex techniques in accordance with their individual needs and desires.

Because of the concentration of the sensual impulses around the area of the clitoris, many women, although unable to reach an orgasm from intercourse, can do so with comparative ease if the clitoral region is stimulated directly. If this is the case, it is advisable for the husband to stimulate the clitoris manually, either during the sex act or, if necessary, even after he has reached his own orgasm. It is often better to bring about a culmination in this manner than to permit the development of a feeling of physical and emotional frustration which sometimes follows an unfulfilled sexual relationship.

Wouldn't such a practice be a perversion, Doctor?

Erotic sex play in marriage is a deviation from the normal only when it serves as the sole means of sexual gratification and comes to be preferred to normal sexual union. As long as it is used merely as a preparation for the sex act or as a means of bringing about its completion and fulfillment, it can hardly be regarded as abnormal. There is nothing perverse or degrading, I would say, in any sex practice which is undertaken for the purpose of promoting a more harmonious sexual adjustment between a husband and a wife in marriage. Of course, aesthetic values and sensitivities have to be considered, and it is important that no sense of impropriety or guilt follow any such conduct, otherwise the effect may be more harmful than beneficial. This, however, is largely a matter of individual judgment and mutual understanding. Two people who are in love and who are emotionally congenial and compatible should not find too much difficulty in adjusting the details of their sexual relationship to their mutual satisfaction.

Do men also differ much in their sex desire and ability?

Yes, in men too there are wide variations in the degree of sex drive and capacity. Some men have strong and frequent sex needs, while others have little desire. According to Kinsey, for instance, for men under thirty years of age the average number of ejaculations, whether following intercourse or other forms of sexual experiences, in 3.3 per week, but there are some men in this age group who have less than one ejaculation per week, and others who have seven or more. These frequencies vary with age, marital status, social and educational level, and constitutional factors.

Sexual Frigidity in Men

Are there men also who are sexually frigid?

Some time ago I published in a popular magazine a short article on sexual frigidity in women. Among the letters which I later received were many from women who complained that not they but their husbands were the frigid ones in their family. Here, as an example, is a paragraph from one of these letters:

Why is it so taken for granted that only women are frigid? In my case it's just the opposite—a husband who is sexually cold, uninterested, and indifferent. Isn't there any help for women with normal but unsatisfied longings who are driven to bitter despair by frigid husbands?

This woman's complaint has much justification. While it is true that frigidity is more frequent among women, it is a condition which is not uncommonly encountered in men too. More often than is generally realized, a woman will complain of her husband's sexual apathy and of his apparent lack of erotic desire. She may accuse him of a loss of affection and even suspect him of infidelity. While in some instances the sexual coldness may indeed be the result of a lack of physical desire for a particular mate, it is more often the expression of an inherently low degree of sexual drive on the part of the man irrespective of the wife he may have.

Sexual Impotence

If a man is sexually frigid, Doctor, does it mean that he will also be impotent?

Not necessarily. The sexually frigid man may still be fairly virile during intercourse, and he may be able to function sexually with considerable competence, but he has little sexual appetite, he is content to go for many weeks or many months without sexual gratification. The impotent man may have very strong and frequent desire, but he cannot achieve a sufficiently firm erection, or else he cannot maintain it long enough to effect penetration.

The general sexual competence of a man, however, depends upon all these factors—the strength of his libido or sexual desire, his ability to have a satisfactory erection, and his capacity to maintain the erection for a sufficient length of time. If this sexual urge is low, if he is incapable of attaining a firm erection, or if he reaches an orgasm too quickly, normal and satisfactory relations may be difficult to achieve in marriage.

Impotence and Marriage

But if a man has little sex desire or lacks adequate potency, why should he want to marry?

In the majority of instances, the man marries without being fully aware of the extent of his inadequacy. It may also happen that the frigidity or impotence develops only after marriage. A man may have had fairly normal sexual experiences before marriage and yet, for various psychological or emotional reasons, find himself sexually inadequate with his wife. Occasionally, a man marries in spite of the knowledge that sexually he is not altogether competent, in the belief or hope that the deficiency will be cured by marriage. This is, of course, a serious mistake. The lack of potency should be remedied beforehand, if possible, and the man should not expect marriage to serve as a cure. At any rate, under such circumstances marriage should not be entered into unless the future wife is fully cognizant of the man's disability and is willing to accept him in spite of his condition. There are men and women, particularly those of somewhat advanced age, who come to look upon marriage merely as a means of establishing a friendship, companionship and a home, and are willing to disregard the sexual factor—but this is a matter for individual understanding and adjustment. They should certainly both have a clear idea of the situation and should be well aware of the potential difficulties which they may encounter in their relations.

Premature Ejaculation

If a man reaches his orgasm very quickly, is it a sign of sexual weakness?

The duration of the act of coitus, as we have already discussed, is subject to wide variations, and men differ greatly in their so-called staying power. Ordinarily the erection should be maintained for many minutes, and the ejaculation should not come for about one or two minutes after intromission, at least not until after some ten, twenty or more coital movements. Some men, however, cannot maintain an erection for even that length of time, and reach their orgasm very rapidly. With men suffering from this disturbance, the ejaculation occurs often immediately upon intromission. In the more severe cases it may even occur as soon as the penis comes into contact with the external genitals of the female, before actual entry has taken place, so that penetration and normal cohabitation are not possible. Disturbances in the sexual function of the male involving rapid ejaculations constitute a rather frequent source of sexual maladjustment and marital disharmony.

Causes of Male Frigidity and Impotence

What causes sexual frigidity or sexual weaknesses in a man?

Well, here again the question which the physician has to determine in each case is whether the condition is physical in origin or whether it is due to psychological factors. In other words, is the man inherently or physiologically low in sexual drive and capacity, or is he merely sexually dormant, as a result of sexual immaturity, inexperience, fear or other causes?

In some instances sexual frigidity or incapacity is the result of hormone deficiencies, local disorders of the sex organs, or other constitutional factors which lead to a diminution of his sexual needs or abilities. Kinsey, for instance, made the significant observation that boys who reach adolescence early in life have a higher intensity of sex desire and a greater total of sexual activity all through life. As the age at which puberty begins depends chiefly on nutritional and inherent constitutional factors, these same factors may perhaps also determine the strength of the man's sexual drive.

In most instances, however, frigidity or sexual incapacity in the male, as in the female, is due to emotional causes. Childhood fixations, overattachment to the mother, fears and anxieties of many kinds, emotional conflicts, neurotic tendencies, latent homosexuality —these and other psychological factors may be the basic cause of a man's sexual apathy or incapacity. "Behind most cases of premature ejaculation lies a fear," says Stekel. Cultural and environmental situations too play an important role. "Sexual incompetence," says Havelock Ellis, "is, to a large extent, a special manifestation of incomplete social adaptation." The pattern of a man's sexual behavior is more or less molded by his childhood experience and training. A man's ideas of what the masculine role should be, his attitude toward women, his religious and social viewpoints, all have a marked effect

on his sexual needs and activities and under certain circumstances
are apt to make him sexually apathetic or inadequate.

Can anything be done to correct or cure sexual weakness?

Yes, indeed. First, it is advisable to obtain competent medical
care, for the treatment will vary with the nature and cause of the
disturbance. Attention to constitutional disorders, the administration of certain hormones and vitamins, local treatment of the genital
tract and other medical measures are at times effective. In many
cases, however, such medical measures are of little value, and main
dependence must be placed upon psychiatric care and guidance.

In the milder forms of rapid ejaculation, it is often possible for
the man to remedy the condition by persistent self-training and control. To avoid reaching a climax immediately after intromission,
the man should attempt to remain quiescent and passive after entry,
without resorting to any coital movements. As the possibility of an
imminent ejaculation passes off, motion may be commenced and
then stopped again before the ejaculation. Deep breathing and a
conscious relaxation of the genital muscles when an ejaculation is
about to occur are helpful. With such intervals of rest it may be
possible to train oneself gradually to maintain the erection for a
longer period and to strengthen the power of sexual control. It is
essential, however, that during these preliminary attempts the wife
should fully cooperate with her husband and, by a sympathetic attitude and either passive or active assistance, give him the necessary
encouragement and help.

Genital Disproportion

*There is one other question in relation to sexual disharmonies that
I should like to ask you, Doctor. Could a lack of proportion between
the male and female organs become a source of sexual difficulties?*

Many people believe that genital disproportions are a frequent
cause of sexual incompatibilities, yet in reality this is but rarely the
case. Only in exceptional instances does a lack of proportion lead
to physical difficulties in intercourse or to sexual maladjustments.
While it is possible, for instance, for the male organ to be so large
as actually to cause pain and discomfort to the woman during coitus,

particularly if she is tense and apprehensive, this is a comparatively rare occurrence. Nor is the smallness of the size of the penis apt to cause serious sexual disharmonies. As a rule, any deficiency in size can be adequately compensated for by a suitable sexual technique. The tissues of the vaginal canal are elastic and distensible and will generally accommodate themselves to the size of the male organ.

When the vaginal walls are very much relaxed and distended, as, for instance, after difficult childbirths, there may be, it is true, a lack of sufficient pressure and some diminution in sexual stimulation and gratification. In modern obstetric practice, however, such relaxations are now being prevented to a considerable extent, or else they are surgically repaired soon after labor. Even if such a condition does exist, a suitable adjustment can still be made. By using her vaginal muscles and learning to tighten and relax them from time to time during the sexual act, the wife can bring about a much closer contact of the genital organs and increase the sensations for both herself and her husband.

But if a man's organ is too small, isn't it likely to affect his sex capacity or his ability to satisfy his wife?

It is not uncommon for a young man to be concerned about the size of his penis, and to fear that it may be too small for satisfactory marital relations. Some carry these fears over into adult life, and they may even avoid marriage or any sexual contacts in order that their deficiency may not be exposed. Yet in reality it is very rare that the male organ is actually too small for adequate functioning.

I recall, for instance, the case of a college graduate twenty-seven years of age, in good health, well developed, intelligent, yet obsessed with the thought that his penis was below normal in size and that he would therefore never be able to enter into satisfactory relations with any woman. Throughout his adolescence his self-consciousness about his supposed deficiency made him avoid any possibility of being seen in the nude by his classmates. He never took a shower in a gymnasium or undressed in the presence of another boy. Yet when he was examined it was found that the dimensions of his penis in both the flaccid and the erect states were even above the average. His fears during all the years of his adolescence and early adulthood were entirely baseless.

Anxieties of this type usually have deep-seated origins. Often they can be traced back to childhood fantasies or experiences. In this particular case, the young man apparently had become anxious about the size of his penis when his father told him that if a boy masturbated his penis would stop growing. As he had masturbated for some years, he was certain that he would never have normal-sized genitals.

Masturbation

You mentioned masturbation, Doctor. Is this practice really so widespread as some say it is?

Well, masturbation, or autoerotism, as it is sometimes called, has been found to be a fairly common sexual practice in nearly all human societies. According to Kinsey's figures, masturbation was resorted to as a sexual outlet by some ninety-two per cent of the men he interviewed, varying somewhat with their social and educational status. Among women the practice is less frequent. They too resort to autoerotic practices, but to a considerably lesser extent than men. It has been estimated that from sixty to seventy per cent of women practice masturbation at one time or another during their lives.

In their study of the sexual behavior of animals and man, Ford and Beach state that in view of the extremely widespread occurrence of self-stimulation of the genitals in animal life generally, masturbation cannot be regarded as "abnormal" or "perverse," but, rather, as a part of the biological tendency of all animals to examine, clean and manipulate the external sex organs. In the course of evolution, with increasing ability to learn and experiment, these reactions have assumed a more frankly sexual purpose and have been used as either a supplement to or a substitute for coitus.

But isn't masturbation harmful? Wouldn't it eventually weaken a person sexually?

There was a time, not so long ago, when practically all kinds of ailments of the body and mind, from acne to insanity, were attributed to masturbation. Today we realize that the dangers have been grossly exaggerated, and that in reality there is little scientific basis for ascribing any dire results to this practice. There is certainly no evidence that it leads to any physical injury or bodily harm.

Any ill effects that may follow masturbation are due in the main to the feelings of anxiety, guilt or self-condemnation which it brings about. Fear of the consequences of masturbation is one of the most common sexual anxieties and constitutes an important sexual problem. Masturbation is generally looked upon as wicked, sinful and abnormal, yet this attitude has apparently not decreased the extent of the practice to any degree. It has merely served to generate in the minds of those who resort to it feelings of remorse and self-reproach, as well as actual fears concerning the possible physical and mental consequences. As a result, most young people who seek release in self-gratification are constantly beset with mental conflicts and anxieties which may seriously affect their social as well as their sexual adjustments.

Let me read to you, as an illustration, a paragraph from a letter which I received some time ago from a young man.

I am convinced that masturbation is an evil which has created havoc in my life. It has sapped my general vitality, it has distorted my sense of intellectual values, and the consciousness of it is a perpetual embarrassment in social contacts. It has now culminated in so complete a destruction of strength, of physical health, of all incentive and zest for living, that suicide, hermitage, or some such refuge often seems inevitable.

This came from a young man of twenty-two who had been masturbating rather moderately for a number of years. A thorough physical examination failed to disclose any evidence of organic trouble, either general or genital. In fact, the man was of fine physique and good intelligence. It soon became evident that his complaints were in no way due to any direct physical effects of his autoerotic practices, but primarily to the fear and anxiety which his preoccupation with the problem had brought about. I may add that he has since married and is now the father of two fine children.

Somewhat similarly, a woman who had not conceived after two years of marriage told me that she was convinced that her sterility was the direct result of masturbation during adolescence, and she was certain that she would remain permanently childless on account of it. There is, of course, absolutely no relation between sterility and masturbation, and, as a matter of fact, this woman conceived readily after a displacement of her uterus was corrected; yet for years the sense of guilt and fear had weighed heavily upon her and had affected both her social behavior and her sexual reactions. "You can hardly realize, Doctor," she told me later on, "what a burden had been lifted off me when I learned that I was not a doomed person because of my youthful acts."

The disturbances, then, which sometimes result from the continued practice of masturbation are basically due to the fears and inner conflicts that are set up, rather than to any actual injury to the sex organs or other bodily structures.

Masturbation and Sexual Adjustment

Well, would masturbation in youth in any way affect the sexual adjustment of a couple later on in marriage?

Not as a rule. Occasionally young people who have practiced self-relief over a long period of time may find it difficult to readjust their sex habits and to derive complete satisfaction from the sex union in marriage. A woman, especially, who during masturbation has achieved her sexual satisfaction only from clitoral stimulation, may later have some difficulty in attaining adequate satisfaction from stimulation during intercourse. Usually, however, the transition from autoerotic to heterosexual experiences is readily attained.

Isn't self-stimulation a rather unsatisfactory and frustrating practice?

Yes, it is an inadequate substitute for more mature satisfactions. It may provide temporary physical relief, but it does not give full emotional gratification, and it often leaves one with a sense of frustration and self-condemnation.

Homosexuality

We have taken a long time today, Doctor, but I would like to ask you a few more questions. Much has been written lately about homo-

sexuality. Are there many people who are sexually attracted to members of their own sex only?

Well, the vast majority of men and women are heterosexual—that is they have sexual desire only for persons of the opposite sex—but there are also some who are exclusively homosexual, with erotic inclinations only toward members of their own sex. According to Kinsey, some ten per cent of all male sexual relationships and a smaller percentage of female relationships are homosexual. Such homosexual behavior has been observed in a great many human societies. It has been found to be more common during adolescence, and to be practiced more frequently by men than by women.

From recent studies it appears that a fairly high percentage of men have both homosexual and heterosexual experiences during the course of their lives. Kinsey states that more than a third of the men interviewed for his study gave a history of some homosexual experiences. This does not mean that all these men were homosexual in the usual sense of the word; only four per cent of them stated that they had remained exclusively homosexual, while another four per cent were nearly so throughout their lives. The others had various amounts of experiences, ranging from a single incident to a considerable number, although most of them were not exclusively or even primarily homosexual for any number of years. Many people, it would seem, are capable of having a variety of sexual responses and can behave either homosexually or heterosexually.

What leads people to become homosexual in their desire and behavior?

First of all it is necessary to distinguish between homosexuality which is merely substitutive, that is, in which a person resorts to homosexual practices because of a lack of opportunity for relations with members of the opposite sex, and homosexuality in which relations with partners of one's own sex are definitely preferred. In our culture there are many situations which may lead a person to accept substitute gratifications in his sex needs. When men or women find themselves segregated for long periods, as in boarding schools, military camps, prisons and so on, homosexual relationships may develop merely as a means of satisfying one's urge for some form of sexual and emotional outlet. Such behavior is sometimes only transient and is usually given up when the person has again an opportunity for heterosexual contacts. However, even under these circumstances some individuals become so conditioned by such experience that they carry on their homosexual interests and develop a preference for this form of sexual behavior.

The causes that lead to the development of preferred homosexuality are not yet clearly understood. At one time it was thought that the condition was physical in origin and that it represented an inborn trait, or that it was due to a disturbance in the balance between the male and female sex hormones in the body. This viewpoint is not accepted now. There is no evidence that constitutional factors or hormonal imbalance play any important part in the development of homosexual tendencies. The administration of sex hormones may affect the frequency and intensity of sex desire and activity, but it does not modify the choice of a partner in sexual relations. The sexual predilections of a person are seemingly determined more by early childhood experiences and by emotional and social influences than by biological factors. Kinsey has even suggested that the persistence of homosexuality throughout human history and in all cultures is due to the fact that this form of sex behavior is an expression of capacities which are basic in the human species. Men and women are apparently able to respond sexually to any adequate stimuli whether they come from persons of the same or the opposite sex.

Would a homosexual experience at one time or another affect a person's sex adjustment later on?

Not necessarily. In fact, some young people become needlessly and unreasonably disturbed because of some isolated homosexual episode. Not so long ago, for example, I saw a boy of twenty who was convinced that he was homosexual because he had had a sexual experience in college with another boy who had approached him for that purpose. He was in constant fear that his behavior might become known to his family and friends, and he was even planning to give up his studies. Several interviews with him showed quite clearly that the homosexual episode was only accidental and not the result of any real homosexual inclinations. Reassured and relieved of his fears, the boy continued with his studies and is now in a professional school. He has since married, and thus far the marriage has been very successful.

Or take the case of a deeply disturbed young college girl who came to see us some time ago. In high school and college she had had several crushes on women teachers and girl schoolmates, but at the time had not associated these with any homosexual tendencies. Later in a course on mental hygiene the instructor had illustrated his lectures with several case histories of sexual deviations. After listening to these discussions the girl felt convinced that she too was a homosexual, and she became seriously concerned. Under the pretext of illness she left college and returned to her home, several hundred miles away, where she later confided her fears to an older sister. A thorough psychiatric study failed to disclose any evidence of homosexuality, and she eventually resumed her studies and her normal life. At present she is engaged to a most personable young man, and I feel confident that she will make a very good adjustment in her marital relations.

I am mentioning these cases only to indicate that homosexual attractions and experiences during adolescence or, for that matter, even in later life, are not evidence of real homosexuality, as it is generally understood. While the number of men, for example, who have had some homosexual experiences during their lives is high, the number who remain exclusively homosexual in their relations is somewhat smaller.

Is it possible to tell a homosexual from his or her appearance?

Only occasionally, and never with certainty. Physically the homosexual may differ in no way from the normal individual. The idea that all male homosexuals have feminine characteristics and that female homosexuals always have a masculine appearance is quite erroneous. The majority of homosexual men and women have the appearance, characteristics and physique of their own sex, and their sexual inclination can be told only from the nature of their reactions and experiences.

Homosexuality and Marriage

But why should homosexuals ever want to marry?

Well, people who have both heterosexual and homosexual inclinations sometimes marry because they feel that they want to establish a normal family relation. Some marry without being fully aware of the extent of their homosexual desires, and some marry in the hope that marriage will change the tendency. Divergent sexual interests, however, usually interfere with a satisfactory marital adjustment. Certainly a homosexual man or woman should not enter marriage merely with the hope that marriage will solve the problems. Whenever a definite homosexual tendency is present, marriage should be undertaken only after careful deliberation and expert professional advice.

We have been discussing all kinds of potential sexual disharmonies, but let me reassure you now that I do not anticipate any difficulties in your own case. From your histories and from the physical findings, I can see no reason at all why you should not make an entirely satisfactory and harmonious adjustment. I have spoken about incompatibilities at such length because I am convinced that ignorance and evasion lie at the base of many marital troubles, and that a frank attitude and adequate knowledge are the best preventive measures.

Next time I intend to discuss with you several aspects of the hygiene of marriage, and I would suggest that in the meantime you make notes of any particular subject that may not have been clear to you in the course of our discussions, and bring the notes with you.

As for books, in addition to those by Ford and Beach, Kinsey, Brown and Kempton, I shall mention a few that are in the main technical in character, but you may wish to have the names for future reference.

Bibliography

Bergler, Edmund, *Counterfeit Sex: Homosexuality, Impotence, Frigidity*, 2nd rev. ed., Grove Press, 1961.

Calderone, Mary S., M.D., *Release from Sexual Tensions*. Random House, 1960.

Dickinson, Robert L., and Beam, Laura, *Single Woman*. Williams and Wilkins, 1949.

Hastings, Donald W., *Impotence and Frigidity*. Little, Brown, 1963. Also in Grove Press and Dell paperbacks.

Hirsch, E. M., *Impotence and Frigidity*. Citadel, 1966.

Kinsey, Alfred C., and others, *Sexual Behavior in the Human Female*. Saunders, 1953. Also in Pocket Books paperback.

Masters, W. H., and Johnson, V. E., *Human Sexual Response*. Little, Brown, 1966.

Stekel, Wilhelm, M.D., *Frigidity in Woman*. Liveright, 1962. Also in Grove Press paperback, 2v.

——, *Impotence in the Male,* rev. ed., Liveright, 1955. Also in Black Cat paperback (Grove Press), 2v., 1965.

CHAPTER IX

HEALTH IN MARRIAGE

As I mentioned last time, I should like to devote today's session mainly to a consideration of several specific problems of sex and reproduction which are related to health in marriage. We have, of course, already dealt with many aspects of marital health, but there are some pertinent questions which we have yet to consider.

You suggested, Doctor, that we should make a note of any particular points we would like you to take up today. We have jotted down several questions about age at marriage, family planning, and sexual adjustments. Perhaps you would like to hear them?

Very well. Suppose we take up your questions, then. For that matter, your notes may coincide with the topics which I myself had intended to discuss with you.

Age for Marriage

First, what is the best age for marriage?

The best age for marriage is the age at which emotional and social maturity is attained. While, biologically, young people may be ready for mating and reproduction somewhere between their sixteenth and eighteenth years, emotionally and socially they may not become sufficiently grown up for the responsibilities of marriage and parenthood until several years later. Chronological age alone cannot, therefore, be taken as the sole criterion of readiness for marriage. The extent of a person's maturity in thinking and behavior is of far greater importance. The economic situation must, of course, also be taken into consideration. In general, however, I would say that the early twenties are the best years for marriage.

Are not marriages taking place later today than formerly?

No, as a matter of fact, during this century there has been a trend in the United States toward earlier marriages. In 1890 the median age at marriage was 22 years for women and 26.1 for men; by 1947 it had declined to 20.5 for women and 23.7 for men. The lowest ages at marriage are generally found in agricultural countries, such as India and China; in industrialized and urbanized countries the average age at marriage rises during the phase of rapid growth, but later it apparently turns down again. As a matter of fact, the chances of marrying at an early age are much greater in the United States than in any other country of the Western world. In 1966 the age for women remained at 20.5, but the age for men was down to 22.8.

It has been suggested that the tendency toward earlier marriage in America at present is due in part to the wider dissemination of contraceptive knowledge which makes it possible for couples to avoid premature childbearing and to plan their families.

What is the legal age for marriage in this country?

The legal age for marriage varies in different states, and it also depends on whether the marriage takes place with or without parental consent. In a few states, girls of twelve and boys of fourteen may marry if their parents consent. In most states, however, the age is sixteen for girls and eighteen for boys when the parents approve; without parental approval the age is usually higher, generally eighteen for girls and twenty-one for boys, although some states require that both partners be twenty-one years of age.

Do differences in age have much influence on the ability of a couple to adjust in marriage?

Statistical studies show that some eighty per cent of men marry women a few years younger than themselves, ten per cent marry women of their own age, and ten per cent marry older women. The chances for a good marriage are generally considered best when the husband is a few years older than the wife. Yet I have seen many happy marriages where the difference in age between husband and wife was considerably greater on either side. The degree of the relative maturity and adaptability of the individuals involved is of more importance than their actual ages.

When marked differences in age do exist, however, a marriage should be entered into only after careful consideration. The man and the woman should have an opportunity to become well acquainted with each other's personality patterns, temperaments, interests, values and ways of living before deciding to marry.

Planning the First Pregnancy

Now, Doctor, about children—how soon after marriage would you advise a couple to plan the first pregnancy?

One can hardly be dogmatic on this point. The ages of husband and wife, their health, their social and economic situation, and their personal preferences would naturally have to be taken into account. As a general rule, I should advise a couple to wait at least one year after marriage before planning a pregnancy. Upon marriage, a man and a woman, often enough with totally different backgrounds, personalities, and habits, are brought together into intimate daily contact. They need time to adjust themselves to each other's temperaments and reactions, to build up their companionship and mutual interests, to strengthen and cement their attachment and affection; they need time to establish their home and their social life; they need time, above all, to prepare themselves economically and emotionally for the task of parenthood. Unless there are some special reasons to the contrary, it is preferable that the first year or so of marital life be free from the many problems which accompany childbearing and child rearing.

Furthermore, even in normal and healthy women pregnancy may sometimes give rise to various temporary physical and emotional indispositions—to nausea, vomiting, nervous irritability, undue sensitivity and so on. If these should occur too soon after marriage, before the husband and the wife have had an opportunity to adjust themselves to each other and to their new mode of life, it may place too great a strain on their relationship and may seriously mar their happiness and affection. It is therefore best to avoid what Margaret Sanger calls "premature parenthood," and the first pregnancy might well be postponed until the second or third year of marriage.

At approximately what age is it best for a woman to have her first baby?

In general, a woman should preferably not have her first child before she is twenty or twenty-one years of age, and not much beyond her thirtieth year. While a girl may become capable of conceiving shortly after she begins to menstruate, the mere onset of menstruation is not a sign of total biological readiness for reproduction. It generally takes several years for adolescence to be completed, and childbearing and child rearing are certainly not advisable until a woman has reached her full physical and emotional development. The age at which biological maturity occurs varies to some degree with race, climate, nutrition and other environmental factors, but in temperate zones a girl is not usually ready for reproduction until she is at least eighteen or, better still, twenty or twenty-one years of age. It is true that in certain Oriental countries marriages often take place at a very early age, even at twelve or thirteen, and pregnancies sometimes occur soon after the onset of puberty. Such a practice, however, appears to be biologically unsound, and for the more northern countries, at least, it would seem that a girl should not conceive, and perhaps even not marry, before she has reached at least the age of eighteen.

On the other hand, while fertility usually lasts until past forty, and while with modern obstetric technique it is quite safe for a woman to give birth even to her first offspring at a rather advanced age, it is nevertheless both medically and socially desirable that a first pregnancy not be postponed much beyond the age of thirty. After the middle thirties fertility normally tends to diminish, and the problems of a first pregnancy, of childbirth and of child rearing at this time are much more involved.

The Size of the Family

What would you consider a desirable number of children for a couple to have?

So many individual factors enter into consideration that it is hardly possible to lay down specific recommendations. The health of the parents, particularly that of the mother, their ages, their social and economic status, their personal predilections and any number of other individual and social factors have to be taken into account. The census report for 1960 showed that in the United States white married women bore on an average approximately 2.5 children, the number varying to a considerable degree with the educational level of the mother. The trend is toward increasingly smaller families. Certainly some couples will want to have at least two or three children, and not many American families can under present conditions plan to have more than four. It is well that the first two babies should come fairly close together, to provide greater companionship for the children and to simplify the problems of their upbringing for the parents. As for later children, whether they should come in close succession or at longer intervals is a matter for individual planning.

If no preventive measures against conception were to be taken, how soon after marriage would a woman conceive?

That would depend primarily upon the reproductive capacity, or fertility, of the particular couple. If both the husband and the wife are highly fertile, conception can occur in the very first month. This, however, is not often the case, and as a rule several months, and sometimes even a year or more, may elapse before the first pregnancy ensues. In his book *Human Sterility,* Meaker makes the following interesting statement on this subject.

When one hundred human couples, young and apparently healthy, marry and have regular intercourse without contraception, the results are easy to predict. In a minority of cases pregnancy will occur immediately, the wife missing her first period. The majority of the wives will become pregnant after delays ranging from a month to a year. In some few cases a pregnancy will appear a year or more after marriage. Approximately ten of the couples will remain childless.

This, of course, is only a statistical average, and, while it may be possible to give such an average for a hundred couples, there is no exact way of telling beforehand how soon after marriage a pregnancy may occur in any particular case.

Contraception and Sexual Adjustment

*Then contraceptive measures must be used from the very begin-
ning if a pregnancy is to be avoided?*

Yes, indeed. If, for health, social, economic or any other reasons,
a pregnancy has to be prevented or postponed for a time, no reliance
should be placed upon the chance that the woman may not conceive
immediately. The very fact that it is possible for conception to follow
a single sexual relation indicates the need for the use of adequate
contraceptive measures from the very first.

It is also advisable to employ contraceptive precautions early in
marriage in order to avoid the recurrent fear and anxiety of an unwanted pregnancy. Such fears are apt to have a very baneful influence upon the marital adjustment of a couple. With many women
the fear becomes an actual phobia which mars every phase of their
marriage. Time and again women have told us that because of the
possibility of an unwanted conception, they had actually discouraged
any tenderness and intimacies on the part of their husbands, and
had made every effort to avoid sexual contact altogether. Let me
read to you a few sentences from a letter which one woman sent us:
"Ever since we were married we were in constant fear and anxiety,
and all the beauty and joy of our love was lost. Our intimate life
became a source of continuous worry to me, and I often dreaded it.
I almost came to look with loathing upon the sexual relation."

Such instances of frustrated and distorted sex lives are not at all
rare. It is obvious that a healthy marriage can hardly exist under
such strains. Neither affection nor tenderness can long survive the
withering effects of continued anxiety and tension. A knowledge of
contraceptive measures can thus contribute materially toward the
health and stability of a marriage.

*Does the type of contraceptive used have any bearing upon sexual
adjustment and satisfaction?*

Yes, the particular method of contraception is sometimes of importance. A man or a woman may respond adequately when one
type is used and yet be unable to react fully when another method
is employed. Many women, for example, have difficulty in reaching

a climax when the husband resorts to withdrawal, yet they will respond completely if a different method is used. Similarly, many men find the sheath a marked deterrent to satisfactory relations and are able to react fully only when the wife is the one to use the necessary protection.

Is Contraception Harmful?

Can the use of contraceptives lead to any injurious effect?

The contraceptive methods which are currently prescribed in planned-parenthood centers and by physicians have been found to be entirely harmless. We have had rather extensive experience in this field and have seen no ill effects from their use. There are, of course, methods which may be harmful; the use of strong chemicals in douches or in chemical contraceptives—these may possibly give rise to local congestions or inflammations, but this does not apply to the approved methods of contraception.

Contraception and Sterility

If a woman uses contraceptive measures for any length of time, will it affect her chances of having children in the future?

The statement is sometimes made that the use of contraceptive precautions may eventually lead to sterility, yet I know of no authoritative evidence to this effect. In his study of human sterility, Meaker states that there is no reason to suppose that sterility will follow the use of approved birth-control measures, and many other authorities have expressed similar opinions. During the course of our work we have had occasion to observe many thousands of women who had employed prescribed contraceptive measures for varying lengths of time, sometimes for many years, and who, when they wished to become pregnant, readily conceived upon discontinuing the contraceptive precautions.

Planned Pregnancies

In a large number of these "planned-pregnancy" cases, we made particular note of the time that elapsed between the abandonment of preventive measures and the onset of pregnancy; in tabulating a thousand records of such planned pregnancies, we found that most of the women conceived within six months, the majority of them, in fact, becoming pregnant during the first or second month after ceasing to employ contraceptive precautions. These findings would indicate that, at least as far as this group of women is concerned, contraceptive measures did not cause any diminution in reproductive capacity, for the fertility of these women was certainly as high as that of women who might never have used any measures for the prevention of conception.

Many women, furthermore, become pregnant very readily when, either through neglect or for some other reason, they omit the use of preventive measures on but a single or a few occasions. This, again, clearly indicates that the resort to contraception does not affect adversely the fertility of a woman. Of course, as we have already seen, over ten per cent of all married couples, whether they ever used contraceptives or not, are infertile, but there is no basis for assuming that this percentage is in any way increased by the use of approved preventive methods.

Vaginal Discharges

Now another question, Doctor. Is it natural for a woman to have a vaginal discharge?

A slight amount of discharge is normally present in the vagina. This comes partly from the cervix, partly from the surface of the vagina itself, and partly from the Bartholin's glands at the entrance to the vagina. Usually, however, this discharge is small in amount, and the woman is hardly conscious of its presence. The discharge may be slightly more profuse just before or just after the menstrual period. A slightly sticky or stringy discharge is also noted by some women at the time of ovulation. If the discharge, however, is continuous and profuse—a condition commonly called "leukorrhea"—it is indicative of some genital irritation or infection which may require medical attention.

Does the presence of a discharge usually indicate a venereal disease?

No, not at all. The vaginal discharge may be caused by a variety of conditions. A frequent cause, for instance, is the presence in the vagina of a microscopic one-celled organism called trichomonas vaginalis, or of a fungus known as monilia. These organisms may affect women who have never had any sexual relations. Just how they get into the vaginal tract is not clearly known as yet, but it is believed that the infection may extend from the intestinal tract into the vagina, or else be in some way introduced from the outside.

These conditions may cause a considerable amount of local discomfort, burning and itching, as well as pain during the sexual relation. Occasionally, the man too may become infected with the trichomonas organism and develop a slight discharge from the urethra, and some burning on urination. In such instances, he may be a source of transmitting the infection to the woman.

Vaginal Douches

Should a woman use vaginal douches for routine cleansing?

Douches need not be used, nor are they required for cleanliness. In fact, normally the vagina is kept in a healthy state through its own physiological processes, and frequent douches may even interfere with this condition.

Vaginal douches should be used only when there is some definite need. When there is a troublesome increase in the normal vaginal secretion, a simple cleansing douche may be employed. One teaspoonful of ordinary salt to a quart of warm water is suitable for such purposes. If the discharge is profuse, medicated solutions may be required, and these will be prescribed by the physician, depending upon the nature of the condition.

Frequency of Intercourse

Now we have a few questions about sex relations in marriage. How often should married people have intercourse, Doctor?

The question of the frequency of intercourse in marriage has long been a subject of inquiry and discussion, and many attempts have been made to lay down rules and regulations. Mahomet, for instance, in the Koran, prescribed a frequency of once a week, but it seems that this applied only to the woman; as the Mohammedan man was permitted more than one wife, he was apparently not bound by these limitations. In the Jewish Talmud a frequency varying from once a week to once a day is advised, depending upon the general state of health and the occupation of the husband. A well-known advice also is that of Luther, who is said to have stated, "Twice a week does harm neither to her nor to me," a suggestion which coincides fairly well with present-day practices.

A number of statistical investigations have been made of the actual frequency of intercourse in marriage. In an inquiry among a thousand married women, made in the 1920s, Katherine Davis found that over seventy per cent reported sexual relations from once to several times a week, twenty per cent less than once weekly, and about ten per cent daily or oftener. In an analysis of ten thousand records from the Margaret Sanger Research Bureau in New York, made in 1933, it was found that eighty-five per cent of the couples had relations from one to three times a week, and only four per cent daily or oftener. A survey of the histories of three thousand women which we later made also showed the average frequency to be between two and three times a week. It is well to remember, however, that these figures apply to couples who had been married for some time. In the early months of marriage the frequency is generally greater and probably approximates the higher figures of once a day or so.

In his survey of sex behavior in the American male, Kinsey found marked variations in the frequency of marital intercourse, depending to a large degree upon the age of the husband. Married men between the ages of twenty-one and twenty-five reported an average of slightly over three relations per week, while those aged thirty-one to thirty-five reported an average of only a little over two relations per week. This frequency steadily diminishes, according to Kinsey's figures, to an average of one and a half times a week for men aged forty-one to forty-five, and to less than one sexual relation a week for men over fifty-six years of age. In each of these age groups, however, there was a great variation in range among the men studied.

It is apparent, therefore, that the frequency of intercourse cannot be prescribed dogmatically, nor is it advisable to institute any routine regularity. Individual sexual capacity and desire, as well as many transitory conditions and circumstances, will normally influence the extent of sexual activity in marriage. Illness, insufficient diet, overwork, emotional strain, will tend to diminish the sexual urge, while rest, a rich diet, erotic stimuli and other factors may temporarily heighten it considerably.

Perhaps the best rule to follow is to permit one's natural desire and capacity to control the frequency of the relations. The physical reaction which follows coitus may serve as a guide in this respect. If one feels greatly fatigued after intercourse or on the following day, a diminution of sexual activity may be advisable. When the coital act, however, is followed by a sense of relaxation and ease, the sexual relations are probably not excessive, and their frequency should then depend entirely upon the desire of the couple.

Frequency and Sexual Compatibility

But if the husband and the wife happen to differ in the degree of their sexual desire, how should they regulate the frequency of their relations?

You have touched upon one of the most pertinent problems in sex adjustment. Marked differences in the sexual urge of the husband and the wife may indeed become a source of sexual difficulties and disharmonies, and it may require a great deal of understanding and sympathy to make a satisfactory adaptation. There are several considerations, however, which should be taken into account.

In the matter of sexual activity, it is the male who is generally the initiator and who takes the more aggressive role. The female is biologically the more passive and receptive, and this passivity is constantly being reinforced in our social life by training, education and convention. While there are some human societies in which both partners are equally aggressive in initiating sexual advances and in the sex act itself, in most cultures the female is expected to assume a passive role in sex relations. Ordinarily, therefore, and certainly at the beginning of marriage, the wife can seldom be expected to take the initiative in the sexual approach, and the frequency of the relation will to a large degree be controlled by the desires of the husband. As a matter of fact, the sexual impulses of a young wife are often latent or dormant, and at first she may hardly even be aware of the extent of her sexual needs and capacities. Her erotic desires may awaken and develop only after the marital relations have been established for some time, and at first, at least, they cannot therefore be taken as a guide for the frequency of intercourse.

There is another reason why the frequency of marital relations will depend largely upon the male. While the woman is able to enter into, or rather submit to, sexual union without any desire at all, the male cannot take part in the sex act unless he has been erotically aroused and has been able to attain an erection. When he lacks desire or is temporarily sexually fatigued, it may not be possible for him to have relations, so that of necessity the husband's capacity will play a large part in determining the frequency of intercourse in marriage.

At the same time, however, the sexual frequency should not be entirely a matter of the husband's choice, but should be adjusted to the responsiveness of the wife and to her reaction to his approaches. The husband should certainly not force his wife when she has definite objections to intercourse, and he should make every effort to choose a time when she is more apt to derive gratification from the union. Nor is it necessary that the husband always be the initiator of the sexual embrace. It is conducive to much greater satisfaction in marriage if every now and then the wife too takes the first step in the sexual approach. A man and a woman who are compatible in other respects, who have a deep affection and sympathy for each other, and who are sexually normal, will, generally speaking, find little difficulty in adjusting the time and frequency of their relations to their mutual harmony and satisfaction. It is important, however, that they be entirely frank in indicating to each other their feelings and desires.

The Rhythm of Sexual Desire

Are a woman's sexual desires greater at certain times than at others?

Yes, there is considerable evidence of the existence of a monthly rhythm in the intensity of the sexual urge of women. The studies of Havelock Ellis, Marie Stopes, Katherine Davis and others seem to indicate that there is a periodic rising and waning of sexual desire during the menstrual month. Our own studies, on a large series of cases, also show a fairly definite rhythm of sex desire in a high percentage of women. Most women state that their erotic impulses are increased either a few days before the onset of the menstrual flow or, more usually, right after menstruation, although the latter rise may be partly due to the abstinence which is generally maintained during the menstrual week. Stopes reported also a second rise of sexual desire at some point in the middle of the menstrual month. There are apparently individual differences in the cycle of desire, and a woman can best determine for herself her own particular rhythm.

Rhythms of Sexual Desire and Fertility

Is there any relation between the fertile period in a woman's cycle and her rhythm of sexual desire?

In animal life there is a very definite relationship between these two cycles. As a matter of fact, the height of sexual desire and the height of fertility coincide. The greatest sexual activity of the female animal manifests itself during the period of rutting, or "heat," which corresponds to the period when the eggs are ripening and are being discharged, and hence when the animal is most likely to conceive. As a result, copulation among lower species occurs only at a time when it is most apt to be fruitful. Among the higher animals, such as the apes, sexual union can occur at any time, but there is also a very definite period during the month when sexual desire and sexual activity are at their highest, and this too corresponds to the time of ovulation and hence of greatest fertility.

In the human female, the relation between the rhythm of fertility and the rhythm of sexual desire is not so apparent. As I mentioned, the increase of sexual desire in the woman is more apt to occur either just before or at the end of the menstrual period, but at these times the woman is least fertile. The second wave of increased desire at about the middle of the menstrual month, which some have reported, would coincide more nearly with the period of greatest fertility in the woman, but these findings have not been substantiated. Perhaps the fact that a woman may desire to have sex relations at times when conception is not likely to result is an indication that for human beings, at least, sexual activity has a specific social and biological value in addition to its reproductive purpose. It has been suggested, in fact, that the readiness of the female to accept the male at almost any time is responsible to some degree for the development of mating and the family among the primates.

Does the male also have a rhythm of sexual desire?

In some species of animals there is a definite periodicity of desire in the male corresponding to that of the female. In these animals the male does not produce any sperm cells at all during certain periods of the year, and his sexual activities are dormant at these times. In the higher species, the male, unlike the female, produces his sex cells continually, and he is therefore capable of impregnating a female at any time. His sexual desires and activities are correspondingly not subject to any seasonal or periodic variations. In man no inherent sexual cycle has been demonstrated. He is, of course, also subject to a certain ebb and flow in his sex needs, but this is apparently due to environmental or general bodily and emotional changes rather than to any specific physiological rhythm.

Would you say, then, that a couple should have relations only at the times of the wife's increased sex desire?

No. It is well for the husband to be aware of the periods of heightened desire on the part of the wife, and he should attempt to some degree, at least, to adapt the marital relations to this rhythm. It is not at all necessary, however, that sex intercourse be limited to these periods. Even if one of the mates has little desire, the mere fact of being a source of gratification to the other may be a highly satisfying experience at times.

Sexual Relations During Menstruation

What about sexual relations during the menstrual period? Would intercourse be harmful then?

There is a considerable divergence of opinion as to the advisability of intercourse during the menstrual period. Formerly a woman was almost universally regarded as taboo during her menses, and sexual relations at this time were strictly forbidden. Among many primitive tribes the woman is even today isolated in a special hut during the days of her menstrual flow, and any article of clothing or food with which she comes into contact is considered contaminated and "unclean." The Bible too prescribed seclusion for the menstruating woman and strictly prohibited any sexual contact with her "as long as she is impure by her uncleanness." Intercourse during the menstrual period has generally been considered both dangerous and sinful.

The sources of these taboos probably lie in the fear of the blood, and the restrictions placed upon the menstruating woman are designed primarily to prevent the menstrual discharge from coming into contact with any object. Incidentally, in an interesting study of human reproduction, Ford points out that the more efficient the methods available to a woman for collecting, concealing and disposing of the menstrual discharge, the less she is isolated or restricted in her activities during this period.

Today we realize, of course, that there is no particular "impurity" about the woman during her menses. It is true that some investigators have found certain toxic substances in the secretions of menstruating women. Nevertheless the fear of contagion from the menstrual discharge is now generally looked upon as merely a survival of primitive superstition. In civilized communities the taboos concerning social contact with women during their menstruation have practically disappeared, and many people have come to look upon sexual relations at this time as neither harmful nor objectionable. It is well to bear in mind, however, that during the days of the menses the sexual organs of the woman are in a state of considerable congestion, and that intercourse at this time may lead to an increase of the menstrual flow and to an aggravation of the discomforts which sometimes accompany this period. Furthermore, if a protective sheath is not used, intercourse during the menses is occasionally followed by a local irritation of the male urethra, due perhaps to the entry of the menstrual secretions into this canal.

Aside from these medical considerations, however, most people consider sexual relations to be aesthetically undesirable during the days of the active flow. Nor is the menstruating woman likely to have much sexual desire. Briffault, in fact, in his book *The Mothers,* makes the interesting suggestion that the menstrual taboo was originally instituted by women themselves, and that it corresponds to the instinctive refusal of female animals to accept the male whenever they are not in a condition for fertile copulation. There are exceptions, of course, and some women do indeed manifest a very strong sexual desire during their menses, or there may be other circumstances which make sexual relations advisable or convenient at this time, but this is a matter for individual consideration and decision. In general, I would say that, while intercourse during the menses may not be harmful, it is preferable to abstain from sexual contact and even from sexual stimulation during the days of active menstrual flow, unless the woman specifically desires it.

Sexual Relations During Pregnancy

After a woman becomes pregnant, for how long is it safe to continue sexual relations?

Among many mammals, as soon as the female conceives she will no longer accept the male, and her sexual activity ceases entirely during the period of pregnancy and sometimes also during the first half of suckling. Among many primitive peoples too, sexual relations are taboo all through pregnancy and even during the nursing period. Briffault suggests that this taboo, as in the case of menstruation, was originally initiated by the woman, and that the primitive human female merely followed biological precedent in imposing a sexual prohibition upon the male during a period when her own sexual instincts were more or less quiescent. Gradually these restrictions assumed a different interpretation and came to be regarded with superstitious awe and fear. Whatever their origin, however, these taboos have long since lost their significance and force in civilized societies, and sexual relations during pregnancy are no longer regarded as either harmful or sinful.

During pregnancy, sex relations should be moderate in frequency and in character. Because of the anatomical changes at this time, the vagina becomes shorter and shallower, and it is necessary to avoid too deep penetration in order not to cause any pressure upon the uterus. Nor should any undue weight be placed upon the woman during this period. This can best be obviated by using the side position, the back position, with both partners lying on their sides, or the cross position for coitus, since these postures are probably the most convenient and comfortable for the childbearing woman.

Today it is generally accepted that if a pregnancy runs a normal course, sexual relations may safely be continued until about the last eight or six weeks before the expected childbirth. Some advise against sexual relations during the few days of each of the first two or three months when the menstrual period would normally have occurred. When there is a history of a previous miscarriage, or when there are staining and cramps which might indicate a threatened miscarriage, sex relations may have to be avoided entirely during the early months of pregnancy, depending, of course, upon the physician's advice in each case. Toward the end of pregnancy sexual relations should be avoided because of the possibility of bringing on labor prematurely.

How soon after the child is born may relations be resumed?

Ordinarily it is advisable to avoid sexual relations for about six weeks following delivery. Primitive taboos against sex relations during pregnancy usually extended also to the period of lactation, and among some peoples sexual relations are prohibited during the entire time that the mother is nursing her baby. As this period sometimes lasted two or three years and even longer, it is evident that there was a long span of abstinence for the woman following conception. The Biblical injunctions are much less severe in this regard. According to the Mosaic laws, a woman is considered "unclean" for forty-one days following childbirth if the child is a son, and for eighty days if the offspring is a girl. Why such a distinction should have been made between the birth of a son and that of a daughter is not quite clear from a physiological standpoint. Nevertheless, the prescribed six-week period of abstinence corresponds closely to present medical opinion on the subject. As I have already mentioned, the generative organs of a woman undergo profound changes during childbearing and delivery, and it takes from five to six weeks after childbirth before they return to their normal condition. During this period it is therefore better to abstain from sex relations, in order to avoid hindering the natural processes of involution.

Sexual Impulse After Menopause

When a woman's menstrual periods cease entirely, I mean when she reaches her "change of life," does she also lose her sexual desire?

Not at all. The cessation of a woman's reproductive capacities does not involve the extinction of her sexual instincts. With advancing years the sexual urge normally tends to diminish, but a woman may continue to have a strong sexual urge for ten, fifteen and even more years after she has reached her menopause. As a matter of fact, a large number of women have an intensification of their erotic impulses during the climacteric, which may in part at least be due to the fact that there is no longer any fear of pregnancy at this time. As a rule, women can continue a moderately satisfactory sex life until well after the age of sixty.

The Male Climacteric

How does age affect the man's sexual capacity, Doctor? Does he too go through a "change of life"?

While some men go through certain physical and emotional changes in their fifties, to which the term "climacteric" has been applied, these are quite different from the "change-of-life" period in women. In the woman, the menopause is characterized by the cessation of menstruation and the loss of reproductive capacity. In the man, there is no sudden cessation of procreative ability, and usually no clear-cut physical or emotional symptoms characteristic of the "change of life."

With advancing age, however, gradually the man too loses his sexual abilities. As he grows older, the strength of his desire and his sexual capacity are progressively diminished. According to Kinsey's figures, the American male is sexually most active during the period of adolescence, between the ages of sixteen and twenty. Thereafter, the sex drive decreases slowly and steadily. For married men between the ages of twenty-one and twenty-five the average frequency of sexual release, through either intercourse, masturbation, or other forms of sexual experience, is about four times per week, but this average gradually drops to only about once a week for men above fifty-six years of age. With increasing age there is also an increase in the amount of time and the amount of stimulation required to produce an erection. This reduction in male sexual activity with advancing age is due mainly to a general decline in physical and physiological capacity, but in part also to social and psychological factors.

Is it true that if a boy is sexually very active in his youth, his sexual capacity will be lessened as he grows older?

There is no scientific evidence that a man's sexual capacities can be used up by frequent sexual activity in youth. On the contrary, there is evidence to show the opposite, that the earlier adolescence and sexual interest begin, the stronger and more frequent the sexual activity of the individual is apt to be in later years. This may be due to the fact that the early onset of puberty is the result of favorable bodily conditions and functions which are conducive to greater sexual activity.

Sexual Continence

There is one other question I should like to ask you, Doctor. Is sexual continence harmful? If the sexual desire is consciously repressed, will it lead to any injurious effects?

If by "continence" you mean the complete avoidance of sexual activity, only a small proportion of people really practice it. It is rarely possible to dam up entirely the stream of the sexual desire; though intercourse may be avoided, other sexual outlets may be used as a source of sex expression. Involuntary nocturnal emissions, masturbation, petting, homosexual practices—these are some of the forms of sex activity which often serve as substitutes for sexual intercourse for both the adolescent and the adult. According to Kinsey's studies, well over ninety per cent of boys become sexually active soon after the onset of adolescence, and they have more sexual experience in one form or another at this age than they do at any later period in their lives. Continence, therefore, as a complete avoidance of any sexual outlet, is practiced by very few men in our society.

If, on the other hand, you mean by "continence" merely the avoidance of intercourse with members of the opposite sex, then its potential effects are open to question. There is perhaps no single problem in sexual physiology and psychology about which there is greater controversy and divergence of opinion. Formerly it was very generally held that even the prolonged avoidance of any sexual relations was altogether harmless. But this opinion may have been based upon what Havelock Ellis calls "an illegitimate mingling of moral and physiological considerations." During the last several decades, particularly since the advent of Freudian psychology, many physicians have come to believe that continued abstinence is not compatible with good physical and mental health and functioning. The fact is that we do not yet possess sufficiently accurate scientific knowledge upon which to base any generalizations concerning the ultimate effects of continued sexual abstinence.

Whether continence might prove harmful in a particular case is a question for individual consideration. Men and women with a strong libido, or those subjected to frequent erotic stimulation, may be considerably more affected emotionally by abstaining from sex relations than those who possess a low degree of sexual desire or lead a cloistered life. Freud remarks that it is a serious injustice that our standards of sexual life are the same for all persons, because, while these standards may be easy for some, they involve the most difficult emotional adjustments for others. I have seen many men and women who showed no evidence of any injurious effects from postponing sexual intercourse until rather late in life, but I have also seen many people who were greatly troubled physically and emotionally by their sexual repressions. It is a matter, therefore, for individual consideration.

Premarital Relations

Would you say, Doctor, that among young people premarital relations are more frequent today than they used to be?

Yes, there is some evidence that there has been an increase in the number of young people who have sexual relations before marriage. This may have come about as a result of a number of medical and social developments which have made premarital relations more feasible and more acceptable. Aside from moral and religious considerations, the major deterrents to sexual relations outside marriage have been, in the words of Dr. Dickinson, three fears, the fears of conception, infection and detection. The first two of these have now been largely eliminated. Modern birth-control methods have greatly diminished the chances of an unwanted conception, and the development of the antibiotics has to a large degree eliminated the dangers of infection. The fear that still remains is the one of detection—that is, of social disapproval. But this too is now gradually lessening. Hence there is today greater freedom in the relations between the sexes.

But doesn't this freedom still apply more to men than to women?

Yes, for the man the problem is, of course, much simpler. Men have generally felt rather free to experiment sexually, and this has long been accepted as a part of our moral code. Kinsey found that more than two thirds of the men he interviewed admitted pre-marital relations, and in certain social strata the percentage was considerably higher.

For the girl, however, the problem is still a difficult one to solve. A large section of our society still regards chastity in a girl as a prerequisite for marriage, and virginity as a necessary quality in a bride. Although the political, economic and cultural emancipation of women has considerably weakened the ideal of premarital chastity, it is nevertheless the woman who has most at stake socially if she decides to enter into a sexual relation before marriage. There is also still the possibility of an unwanted conception. Through carelessness or the ineffectiveness of contraceptive measures pregnancies do occur in spite of their use. It is difficult enough when a married woman conceives unwillingly and accidentally, but it is a much more serious problem in our culture if a pregnancy occurs before marriage.

But if, as you said, men and women mature so much earlier sexually than they do socially, what solution can they find for their sexual needs?

In societies where marriage takes place at an early age, sexual relations begin very soon after biological maturity is reached. In our culture, however, we are faced with a difficult situation. Early marriage is not feasible, because of social and economic circumstances, while moral, ethical, religious and legal standards frown upon sex relations outside wedlock. At the same time, however, sex is constantly exploited commercially and sex desire stimulated by a wide variety of means—by the theater, the film, the popular story and picture magazine, the newspaper and commercial advertising. Young people are thus subjected to recurrent stimulation and suppression, to arousal and restriction, a situation which often plays havoc with their physical and emotional stability.

A variety of suggestions have been made to meet the situation. Some people maintain that premarital chastity is socially and morally necessary and should be preserved at all costs. Abstinence until marriage, they say, is not only desirable on religious and ethical grounds but is also beneficial because it strengthens will and character and contributes to personal development and achievement. Some advocate a return to early marriage or the adoption of some other form of socially approved sexual alliance for young people, a relationship which would be legally sanctioned but which at the beginning would not imply permanence or involve full economic responsibility; such a union would automatically assume all aspects of a permanent marriage at the expiration of a specified length of time or the occurrence of a pregnancy. There are others who hold that the sexual behavior of adults should not be subject to social or religious control, and they favor the easing of present-day restrictions and greater freedom of sex expression.

None of these solutions, however, is really satisfactory or meets present-day needs. We must frankly admit that no socially sanctioned solution to the problem of the sex needs of young people has yet been found.

What is your opinion, Doctor, about premarital relations?

It is well to bear in mind that the sexual relation is not merely an individual matter; it involves the rights and privileges of another person and carries with it many social implications. A certain degree of social control over sex activity is therefore desirable and is found in practically every human society. Certainly as long as our present moral standards prevail complete freedom of sex expression is hardly feasible. The violation of accepted morals and mores, particularly if it is done furtively and secretively, often proves more disturbing to personality and emotional balance than the conscious suppression of the sexual impulse. One may intellectually feel free from conventional attitudes, yet emotionally remain tied to them. The basic conflict between biology and culture, between desire and inhibition, must be resolved individually in each instance.

Complete sexual freedom does not offer an adequate solution to the problem of sex needs during youth. The sexual union is not only a physical contact; it is an emotional relationship as well. It is this aspect of sex life, as a matter of fact, which brings the greatest joy and satisfaction in human relations, a type of satisfaction which can hardly be achieved in casual sexual relations.

Sexual promiscuity is certainly undesirable. It may bring a transient physical satisfaction, but not a deep emotional fulfillment. In spite of our changing values, a lasting union of one man with one woman is still the most ideal form of human sex relationship.

Ideal Marriage

What would you consider a happy or ideal marriage?

An ideal marriage, I would say, is one that meets most adequately the essential objects of the marital union. If you will recall, I mentioned during our very first session that I consider the main purposes of marriage to be companionship, sexual intimacy and the establishment of a family. In other words, marriage is based upon the need for being and living together and the emotional security this provides, upon the need for sexual expression, and upon the desire for the begetting of offspring; an ideal union is one that fulfills most effectively these several requirements.

Obviously, a true friendship and companionship can be present only where there is a compatibility of intellect, of temperament, of interests, of tastes, and above all a mutual affection and attraction. Love is, in fact, one of the essential elements in any marriage. "I would just as soon attempt to bind two stones together without cement," said John Haynes Holmes once, "as to bind two lives together without love." There is some tendency nowadays, it is true, to look upon love as a mere survival of a sentimental era, yet even so realistic a philosopher as Bertrand Russell maintains that there is something of inestimable value in the relations of a man and a woman who love each other with passion, imagination and tenderness, and he adds that to be ignorant of this love "is a great misfortune to any human being." Indeed, ideal marriage is hardly possible without such mutual love and affection.

The importance of a satisfactory sexual adjustment to the achievement of happiness in marriage we have already discussed on several occasions. Conjugal affection should have a strong element of passion mixed with it. Havelock Ellis defines love as "a synthesis of lust and friendship," and both of these are necessary to the establishment of a happy marriage. Intelligent sex education during youth and adolescence, an adequate premarital preparation and the cultivation of an art of sexual love are valuable aids toward marital harmony.

Lastly, the marriage must eventually grow into a family, and the mates become parents. "The fullness of love cannot come without children," writes Will Durant, and he stresses the fact that marriage was designed not so much to unite mate with mate as to unite parents with children. While a childless marriage may be quite happy, it is the coming of offspring that brings complete fulfillment to a marriage. This implies, of course, physical and eugenic fitness for procreation on the part of both husband and wife.

There is one other element in marriage that should be mentioned, although it does not come directly within the scope of our discussion, and that is the importance of social and economic security to happiness in marriage. Again and again we come across marital dissension, discords and maladjustments which are caused not by a lack of affection, nor by sexual incompatibility or reproductive incapacity, but by a lack of the necessities of life, by poverty and economic insecurity. A striking indictment of our society is the very fact that so many young people must postpone marriage for years because of economic uncertainty, or must postpone childbearing because they cannot afford the luxury of a child. Under such circumstances it is obviously difficult to realize happiness in wedlock. Perhaps a better social order will eventually make also for more satisfactory and happy marriages.

Our next session will be the last one. I am planning to discuss with you then some of the elements that go into the making of a successful marriage. In the meantime you may perhaps wish to read some books dealing with the question of marital happiness, and I shall therefore mention a few now.

Bibliography

Burgess, Ernest W., and others, *Courtship, Engagement and Marriage*. Lippincott, 1954.

Ellis, Havelock, *Sex and Marriage*. Random House, 1952.

Fishbein, Morris, and Kennedy, R. J. R., *Modern Marriage and Family Living*, rev. ed. Doubleday, 1955.

Fromme, Allan, M.D., *Ability to Love*. Farrar, Straus, 1965. Also in Pocket Books paperback.

——, *Sex and Marriage*. Everyday Handbook Series paperback (Barnes and Noble), 1967.

Groves, Ernest R., *Preparation for Marriage*. Emerson, 1944.

——, and others, *Sex Fulfillment in Marriage*. Emerson, 1943.

Himes, Norman E., and Taylor, Donald L., *Your Marriage*, rev. ed. Holt, Rinehart and Winston, 1955.

Landis, Judson T., and Mary G., *Building a Successful Marriage*, 4th ed. Prentice-Hall, 1963.

——, *Personal Adjustment, Marriage and Family Living*, 4th ed. Prentice-Hall, 1966.

Levy, John, M.D., and Munroe, Ruth. *The Happy Family*, Knopf, 1938. Also in paperback.

Peterson, James A., *Toward a Successful Marriage*. Scribner's, 1960.

CHAPTER X

HAPPINESS IN MARRIAGE

This will be our last session together, and I have planned to devote it to a discussion of several factors that contribute to the happiness and success of marriage. Let us review briefly some of the elements that enter into the making of a happy marriage and a happy family.

You may recall that in speaking of the motives for marriage I mentioned that the chief satisfactions which people seek in the marital relation are the security of an enduring affection and companionship, a satisfying sexual relation and the building of a home and a family. During the course of our conversations, we have talked in considerable detail about the sexual and reproductive elements in marriage. Today I want to dwell largely on the social and psychological factors which affect the stability of marriage and the family in our culture.

Current Marital Instability

I am glad that you are bringing these questions up, Doctor. We were talking only the other day about the reasons why family life seems to be so much less stable now than it used to be.

Well, the current instability of marriage and the family is the result of many social and cultural changes. These changes have occurred so rapidly that they have as yet not been fully absorbed into our way of life. The tremendous growth of the factory and industry, the continuing migration of people from the country to the city, their mobility and frequent change of residence, the entry of women into industry, the changing economic roles of husband and wife, the transition from a patriarchal to a democratic form of family life—these and many other economic and cultural factors have affected greatly the functions and the structure of the family. This, in turn, has led, for the present at least, to greater family instability.

Changing Family Functions

In what way are the functions of the family different today from what they used to be?

For one thing, the family of today is no longer the economic self-sufficient unit it formerly was. The members of a family do not work together, and an increasing proportion of married women engage in occupations outside the home. Nor is the family today the major center for the education, recreation or protection of its members. Formerly the home was the factory, the schoolhouse, the playground, the hospital. People were born, bred and educated in the home, and they worked, lived and died within the family unit. Today many of the family's social functions are being taken over by communal or commercial agencies. The functions as well as the form of the family are changing to conform with these new cultural conditions.

What, then, are the functions of marriage and the family in our present-day society?

The family today is in a stage of transition. It is changing from the older patriarchal and authoritarian system to a newer democratic and companionship form. In this new type of family the emphasis is primarily upon the intimate interpersonal association between husband and wife, parents and children. As the institutional functions of the family diminish, the personal relationships within the family unit increase in significance.

In our modern society the chief functions of marriage and the family are to provide a center for affection and emotional security, for sex satisfaction and procreation, and also for the transfer of the cultural heritage from one generation to another. The family remains as a rock of refuge, a sanctuary to which people still turn for protection and security. "In times of social flux," wrote Ernest Groves, a keen social observer, "the family becomes more than ever the final refuge for those who can find little sense of security elsewhere." Only within the framework of marriage and the family can a man and a woman best develop the full sense of togetherness, of belonging, of interdependence, which is basic to the growth and development of their own personalities. The social functions of the family may be diminishing, but there is an increasing emphasis on the emotional satisfactions, on the intimate interpersonal associations, which marriage and the family provide.

The family also retains its fundamental functions of procreation and child care. It provides a socially sanctioned unit for the production of children, and the most suitable environment for their physical and emotional development. The paramount importance of parental affection and care for the emotional growth of the child and the development of its total personality is constantly stressed by modern psychiatry. The family unit remains, then, as the basic cultural and socializing factor in human development.

Marital Conflicts

But doesn't the fact that there are so many marital troubles today and that so many marriages break up and end in divorce show that marriages are less happy now than they used to be?

Not necessarily. Marital conflicts are not new. Even Adam and Eve had their difficulties in the Garden of Eden. From time immemorial, husbands and wives have disagreed and quarreled and made up. Formerly, however, marriages and families were held together, in spite of such conflicts, by external adhesive forces—the forces of religion, of law, of social pressure. Today these outer forces are no longer able to sustain an unstable marriage. To survive, the family must possess inner forces, inner resources, an inner unity and cohesion between husband and wife, parents and children.

The increasing number of divorces may, as a matter of fact, merely indicate that we demand more of marriage today than we did a generation or two ago. Nimkoff has made the interesting point that just as the marked increase in the number of hospital patients does not necessarily mean that there is more sickness today than in times past, but signifies only that facilities or hospitalization have increased and that people are more willing to make use of them, so the growth in the number of divorces may mean only that people are more ready to accept radical procedures in instances of marital illness. The family, then, is really not disintegrating, it is merely adapting itself to the new social trends.

Causes of Marital Conflicts

What would you say are chief causes of conflict in marriage today?

Marital discords may stem from many sources. Perhaps we can divide them into three major categories. First, conflicts may arise because either the husband or the wife or both are emotionally immature, or unstable, or have neurotic personality disturbances which keep them from a satisfactory adjustment to each other. Second, they may be due to the fact that the particular couple are not well mated. There may be marked differences in their attitudes, values and interests; they may not have enough love for each other; their sex life may be unsatisfactory; or some serious childbearing problem may exist. Third, conflicts may be caused by outside influences —social, economic, parental—any one of which may hamper the development of a good relationship between husband and wife. In other words, the source of marital conflicts may lie either in the personalities involved or in the marriage itself or in the environment. It is not, of course, always possible to isolate the exact cause or to place it in one particular category, for often a number of factors play a part, and they become closely interrelated and interwoven.

Temperamental Compatibility

You mentioned the personality factors first. Would you say that this is of major importance in the ability of a couple to get along together?

Yes, quite so. The success or failure of a marriage depends to a very large degree upon the personalities of the husband and the wife. The character and temperament of the couple, their disposition and patterns of behavior, the maturity of their thinking and actions— these are perhaps of the greatest importance in the making or breaking of a marriage. You may recall, perhaps, that in our first discussion I mentioned the fact that some people are emotionally not fit for marriage. People with neurotic personalities or psychopathic tendencies find it difficult to make a good adjustment in any human relationship, and especially so in marriage, which requires the closest type of intimacy in daily life. When such people marry they carry over their neurotic form of behavior into their marital association. The girl, for example, who is strongly tied to her parents, who lacks self-reliance and "runs home" at the slightest disagreement with her husband, or the man who flies into a rage when he meets any obstacles to his wishes, or who escapes his responsibilities or his feeling of inadequacy by resorting to alcohol, is not likely to make an easy adjustment in any marriage. The problem then lies in the personalities involved rather than in the marriage itself.

But does not marriage sometimes change the personality of an individual?

Yes, it is true that with marriage a new relationship is established which in itself influences the behavior patterns of husband and wife, and some people grow and mature in the warm, secure and stimulating climate of a marital relationship. Yet, in the main, men and women bring into marriage a fairly fixed personality structure, and after marriage they are likely to act in a manner similar to the way they acted before marriage.

Some studies have shown that men and women who are kindly and friendly, cooperative and tolerant in their social behavior are more likely to make good husbands and wives in marriage. This is presumably due to the fact that they carry over these characteristics into their home and family relation. On the other hand, the man who is irresponsible or domineering in single life will continue to be the same after marriage, and the girl who is demanding or intolerant before marriage is likely to carry the same traits into her marital relations. A husband, therefore, who expects to remold his wife to his tastes and patterns of conduct, or the wife who marries a man with expectations that she will reform him or change him to her liking, is apt to meet with considerable disappointment.

On this question of personality and marriage, let me quote a statement from Terman, who has made a careful study of the psychological factors in marital happiness. "Whether by nature or nurture," he writes, "there are persons so lacking in the qualities which make for compatibility, that they would be incapable of finding happiness in any marriage. There are others less extreme who could find it only under the most favorable circumstances, and still others whose dispositions and outlook upon life would prevent them from acute unhappiness however unfortunately they are mated." In other words, the personalities of husband and wife, their disposition, their emotional maturity, are of prime importance in determining their chances of happiness in marriage. The kind of marriage a person will make depends first upon the kind of person he is, and second upon the kind of person he marries.

Emotional Maturity

You speak of emotional maturity as an important element in a successful marriage. What really do you mean by emotional maturity?

Well, maturity means being grown up. A child is obviously immature—physically, mentally, emotionally. A child cannot walk alone, in both a literal and a figurative sense; it is dependent on others for the satisfaction of its needs, for support and guidance. Nor can a child think logically or rationally, or have much control over its expressions and actions. With the years there generally come added bodily strength, physical independence, greater intellectual ability, increased emotional development—an ability to act and react with physical and emotional control. Some children fail to grow up physically and remain weak and stunted; some fail to develop intellectually and are mentally deficient; and some remain emotionally undeveloped and immature. "When I was a child," Saint Paul wrote to the Corinthians, "I spake as a child, I understood as a child, I thought as a child; but when I became a man, I put away childish things." But many people never grow up fully. In their thinking, in their feeling, and in their actions they continue to be "as a child."

Signs of Maturity

Is there any way, though, of telling whether a person is emotionally grown up?

Very well, let us consider some of the signs of maturity. A mature person has, first of all, shall we say, insight and foresight in his thinking. He can evaluate himself as well as the world around him in a realistic manner. When we are young we often live in a world of fantasy, of unreality; we picture ourselves to be the chosen one, the Prince Charming, the hero, or else the rejected, the despised, the ugly duckling. As we grow up, we gradually learn to understand ourselves better, to evaluate ourselves as we actually are. We come to know our strengths and weaknesses, our abilities and disabilities. We gain insight into our thinking, our feeling and our behavior.

As we grow up we also develop foresight. We learn to face realistically the facts of life and to anticipate the results of our actions. We learn to foresee the possible consequences of our behavior. We no longer permit our desires to dominate completely our thinking or actions.

Emotionally, a mature person develops a sense of independence. When we grow up we can stand by ourselves. We are able to make our own judgments and decisions. The dependent person lacks a sense of security; he lacks confidence in his own abilities. He therefore tends to lean on other people, he looks to someone else for support and protection. The mature individual is self-reliant and assumes responsibility for his behavior. Nor does he escape reality by turning to daydreams, to fantasy or to artificial means of sedation or stimulation.

Another sign of being grown up emotionally is the ability to show and to share love and affection, to actually "care for" someone. In infancy and childhood the feeling of love is basically self-centered. A child wants things for itself, to satisfy its own desires and needs. The child has little feeling for giving or sharing with someone else. The love of a mature person, however, is of a different quality. There is a genuine desire to share with another person, to share thoughts, feelings and possessions. There is the desire not only to be happy but to give happiness, not only to obtain satisfaction but to give satisfaction to a beloved person. This is the kind of love, incidentally, that is essential for a successful marital relation.

Mature thinking and feeling express themselves in mature actions and behavior. A child is likely to act reflexively; an adult, reflectively. The child is impulsive in its actions—he runs after the ball in the middle of the street without thought of the potential dangers; an adult's reactions are more deliberate—he recognizes hazards and will change his actions accordingly. In his behavior the mature person shows both flexibility and control. He is neither rigid nor compulsive, but adapts his action to the situation. He can accept authority and discipline as well as responsibility and power. He learns to cooperate with other people, to make the necessary adjustments and adaptations in life.

Why is it that people differ so much in character and in the degree of their maturity?

Well, no two individuals are really alike. They differ from each other in physique, in intelligence and in emotional reactions. Our bodies and our minds are what they are as a result of nature and nurture, of the constitutional qualities which we inherit from our parents and of the environmental factors which have molded us during the course of our life. Similarly, the differences in our personalities, in our feelings and attitudes, are partly the result of inherited constitutional factors and partly the result of the psychological and social conditioning to which we have been exposed from infancy. As these environmental factors differ of necessity from individual to individual, so do our attitudes and behavior patterns vary. A child, for example, brought up in an atmosphere of love and protection develops a sense of being wanted, of belonging, of security, while a child brought up in an indifferent or hostile environment may never acquire these feelings. Many of the feelings and attitudes which men and women acquire during their formative years are carried over into maturity, and these influence the personality of the individual and the type of adjustment he makes in his marriage and in his life.

It would seem to me, though, Doctor, that it is rather difficult to live up to the criteria you mentioned, and to achieve full maturity.

Yes, you are quite right. Most of us show evidences of immaturities of one kind or another. We are all likely to revert at times to childish forms of thinking or behavior, the result perhaps of our childhood experiences and the tensions and insecurities of our present-day life. If, however, we try to understand the signs and the causes of occasional immature actions and reactions on our part and on the part of our mate, we can become more tolerant and acceptive. This in itself is evidence of being grown up. As for the future, better parental understanding, guidance and care and a more stable social order should lead to greater general maturity in the generations to come.

Cultural Compatibility

But suppose both the man and the woman have what you may call normal or mature personalities, but they come from different backgrounds or differ in their education, or in their interests, or, let us say, in their politics. Would that be a serious obstacle to a successful marriage?

Well, differences of this kind, as I mentioned before, form a second major source of marital conflicts. A husband and wife may be fairly stable and well-balanced individuals, but if they differ widely in cultural background, in viewpoints and tastes, in social standards or ethical values, in their "way of life," they are likely to come into frequent conflict and will find a good adjustment more difficult to attain. They will be culturally incompatible. Let me illustrate this point with the history of a couple, let us call them John and Mary, whom I saw not long ago.

John and Mary came in together for a consultation because they were very much disturbed about their constant quarrels and disagreements. John was twenty-nine and Mary twenty-five, and they had been married for nine months. John came from a large, patriarchal Italian family and was brought up in an Italian household and way of life. There were seven children in the family, and all of them were dominated by the father. The children had very little freedom, and the sisters, especially, were kept under strict discipline and were seldom permitted to go out alone or to meet anyone without constant supervision. Mary, on the other hand, was a Canadian girl, one of two children, brought up in a democratic home where there was much equality and sharing between father and mother, and great freedom for their children. She developed a strong independent will of her own, and a mature attitude toward her role as a woman and a wife.

John and Mary met at a party, fell in love, and were married within six months. Yet soon after marriage the differences in their cultural backgrounds and attitudes toward family life began to manifest themselves and proved to be a source of frequent disagreement. John was very possessive and jealous. He wanted Mary to stay at home while he was at work, he resented her going out of the house even with her girl friends, he felt that as a husband he was the master of the house and that she should submit entirely to his wishes; he also did not want her to use any contraceptive measures and insisted that she plan a pregnancy within the first few months after marriage. Mary rebelled against his attempts at domination. She wanted to make her own decisions and lead a more independent life; she wanted to be free to visit her friends and to go out with them at times, and she wanted to wait at least a year before planning a baby. These differences in attitudes were the cause of increasing discord in their marriage.

It was only after they began to obtain some insight into the reasons for their conflicts, the marked differences in their family cultures, in their needs and expectations in marriage, that they were able to make the necessary compromises in their daily life. They recognized, too, that because of these differences they had lost sight of the major values of married life which both of them shared quite equally. They developed a greater tolerance for each other's attitudes and views and eventually made a successful adjustment in their marriage.

Such difficulties are in part the result of the greater complexity of the American culture in our present era. In this country more than anywhere else we find a wide mixture of races and nationalities and an extensive migration of peoples from one area to another. This has led to greater mingling of divergent cultures, and to marriage between people of different characters and patterns of life. As a result we find more frequent marital conflicts in American marriages during this transitional stage.

Would you say, then, that people coming from different social or cultural backgrounds should not marry?

No, not at all. Here again it would depend largely upon how mature and how personally adjusted the two of them are. If a husband and wife can and will respect and accept each other for the kind of person each is, without always trying to recast the mate into one's own particular mold, or have the other "give in," they may get along very well. I have seen many marriages between people of vastly different backgrounds, social status, political views and educational level which were highly successful.

Interfaith Marriages

But if a couple belong to different religions, what are their chances for a successful marriage?

The chances for the success of a so-called interfaith or mixed marriage would depend above all upon the ability of the couple to face the situation maturely and realistically. If they decide to marry merely because they are romantically in love and feel attracted to each other, without a clear evaluation of the potential hazards they may have to overcome, they are likely to meet with serious difficulties in their marriage.

It is not so much a question of the different faiths to which they belong as their general attitudes toward the dogmas of their particular church. If both the husband and the wife are understanding and tolerant and have no desire to impose their own religious beliefs on their mate, they may get along very well. But if one or the other is fanatical about his own faith, it may be difficult for them to achieve a satisfactory adjustment. As a matter of fact, conflicts on religious dogma may be even less important than disagreements about the problems of everyday living which result from religious differences. Such questions as church attendance, the religion to which the children shall belong, the type of education they shall receive, the use of birth-control measures, tensions between in-laws, may loom up large as a source of continuous irritations.

Sometimes, too, a person may believe that he has completely freed himself from religious prejudices, yet, under the stresses that come up in marriage, these prejudices may unexpectedly emerge from hidden recesses and manifest themselves in some unfortunate manner. People who have harbored deep prejudices against members of other faiths should therefore realistically evaluate their feeling before entering into a mixed marriage.

However, if a man and a woman from different religions come to marriage with a clear understanding of the many obstacles they are likely to encounter and of the numerous adjustments that will have to be made, and if they are flexible enough in their behavior to make these adjustments, their marriage may be very successful.

Isn't it true, though, Doctor, that people with very similar backgrounds and interests may not get along well because they are not suited to each other?

Yes, indeed. A man and a woman may be of the same culture and the same faith, and have similar tastes and ways of life, yet they may not be happy together because the marriage fails to provide them with the basic satisfactions which people seek in the marital relation. As I have already mentioned several times, in marriage people look for the security of love and companionship, for sexual fulfillment and for the building of a home and a family. A man and a woman who are good companions, good sexual partners and good parents are thrice blessed. But these blessings do not come to all in equal measure. In one or more areas the marriage may fail to meet the basic needs and expectations.

Economic Factors in Marriage

What about economic factors? Don't many troubles in marriage come from that source?

Yes, they do. These belong to the third category of marital problems—those due to the outside sources. You will recall, perhaps, that in our first session we spoke of economic fitness for marriage, and I pointed out that in all human societies the husband is the provider and the wife the preparer. In our culture these economic roles in the family are changing rapidly, and the basic pattern of the economic interrelationship of the sexes is breaking down. The stresses and strains caused by these changes, as well as by the social uncertainties of our time, are indeed a frequent cause of family disagreements and quarrels. A husband and wife may both be well-balanced and mature, they may be congenial and compatible in their interests and ways of life, and they may be well-adjusted emotionally and sexually, yet external social factors, such as economic insecurity, unemployment, housing shortages, may lead to serious marital rifts.

The importance of social and economic security to happiness in marriage can hardly be overstressed. The fears and anxieties that come from economic insecurity are often transferred to the home and make husband and wife irritable and impatient with each other. Nevertheless, even here the degree of the adjustment will depend upon the personality traits of husband and wife. Greater income does not always make for greater marital satisfaction. Far more important are the personalities of the couple and their ability to make a good adjustment in the face of social and economic difficulties.

Parents-in-Law

Would you put in-law troubles in the same category? From discussions with our friends we gather that interference by the parents-in-law may be a serious hazard to the development of a good marriage.

Yes, in-law situations are a frequent source of marital conflicts. They can become a serious handicap to a young couple who are attempting to establish a satisfactory marital relationship.

Parent-in-law difficulties really stem from two sources. They result from the failure of one or both of the partners to give up their emotional dependence upon their parents, or from the failure of the parents to relinquish their hold upon their grown-up children.

Many young people remain tied to Mother's apronstrings even after they grow up. They do not attain sufficient self-reliance to function adequately by themselves. When they marry they continue to look to their parents for emotional support. When difficulties arise in their marriage they "run home" for sympathy, or advice, or aid.

Recently, for example, a young husband told me with deep resentment of his wife's complete dependence upon her mother. When they were first married, the wife persuaded him to live with her parents for a time. Later, when they finally decided to move to an apartment of their own, the wife insisted that it be near her parents' home. Mother-in-law chose the furniture for their home, she shopped for the linens and the dishes, and she even accompanied her daughter to the grocery for the daily purchases. Whenever any kind of domestic problem arose in their home life, the wife, instead of discussing it with her husband, would run to Mother for advice. What irked him most, however, was his finding that the mother-in-law even had a latchkey to their apartment and could come in at any time.

The wife was an only child who had been overprotected by the parents throughout her life and was still totally dependent upon her mother emotionally. Only after a number of discussions did she become aware of the nature of her relationship to her mother. Eventually she was able to gain sufficient strength to relinquish her childhood dependence and assume her role as a wife in her own family.

In other instances the parents are the ones who fail to relinquish their dependency on the children and continue to hold on to them even after they have left the parental home. They dominate the young couple, impose their own values and standards upon them and prevent them from developing an independent family life of their own. In such cases parental domination may be a source of many marital conflicts.

Do you feel, then, that a young couple should avoid making their home with their in-laws?

If possible they should preferably make their own home. Among some peoples, it is true, especially where the patriarchal form of family life prevails, newly married couples usually remain with either the husband's or the wife's parents for many years. This is their accepted way of life and may therefore call forth little friction or resentment. In our culture, however, where the family is organized on a democratic basis, married couples expect considerable independence and privacy, and parental interference may become a source of serious marital disturbance. Whenever possible, young couples should live by themselves. They should have the opportunity to make their own adjustments without being subject to constant parental supervision and guidance. Living by themselves, they will better be able to assume their full responsibilities in the marriage and their respective roles as husband and wife.

What does the success of a marriage depend on, Doctor?

As I see it, the success or failure of a marriage depends upon the three factors which we have already discussed in connection with marital conflicts. One is the respective personalities of the husband

and the wife, the degree of their emotional maturity, their balance and stability. The second is the extent to which the two are mutually compatible and congenial in their interests, their tastes and their ways of life, as well as the extent to which the marriage meets their basic individual needs for love and companionship, for sex satisfaction and for the building of a family. The third involves outside influences—economic security, social adjustments, satisfactory family relations. These three factors often interact so that in actuality there are usually multiple causes which enter into the making of the quality of a marriage.

Predicting Marital Success

Is it possible to predict beforehand the chances of success for a particular marriage? I mean, are there any tests that a couple could take before they marry to find out whether their marriage can be successful?

A number of able investigators have in recent years attempted to develop tests which would appraise the marital chances of a couple. First they developed criteria for rating marriages as being either happy or unhappy, and then they obtained a great deal of information about the backgrounds and personalities of the husband and wife, and correlated these findings with the degree of marital success of the couple. They studied their respective home environments, their ages, education and occupations, the length of their acquaintance prior to marriage, their health status, their attitudes on religion, sex, children and so on, and they also studied their personality traits. On the basis of these factors they attempted to determine which qualities made for good and which for bad marriages.

These investigations are of much interest. Some believe that with the aid of such studies it is even now possible to predict the future progress of a marriage with some degree of probability. However, it seems to me that, for the present at least, marital-prediction tests should be regarded as being only in the experimental stage. Their main limitation is that such tests apply to the group within which the individual falls, rather than to the individual himself. With further research, however, marital-prediction tests may become a useful social measure.

Preparation for Marriage

If a boy or a girl were to ask you, Doctor, for suggestions that might help them make a good marriage later on in life, what would you tell them?

There are two main steps, it seems to me, that would help young people achieve greater happiness in their marriage.

The first is: *Prepare yourself for marriage.* Men and women are educated and trained today for all types of occupations, trades and professions, but not for the one job which will play the most important role in their life—that of marriage and parenthood.

The basic preparation for marriage is to know and understand oneself. The quality of a marriage depends upon two factors— upon anatomy and attitude. For successful living in marriage, it is desirable to have some knowledge of both the human body and human emotions. The more a person understands the fundamental facts of the structure and function of sex and the reproductive organs, the more likely he is to make a good physical adjustment in marriage. Similarly, the more aware he is of his own and his mate's attitudes toward marriage and family living, the more he understands the factors that motivate human behavior, and the more insight he has into the ways and the whys of his thinking and feeling, the more apt he will be to make a good personal and emotional adjustment in the family unit.

When should preparation for marriage begin?

Education and preparation for marriage are really a continuous process. Marriage preparation is, in fact, a part of everyday education for living. Since many of our attitudes toward marriage and the family are formed early in life, education for marriage actually begins in infancy, in the parental home, and it continues well into maturity. Children develop attitudes and values long before they can even understand the physical facts of life. Hence, the formation of sound attitudes in childhood may be even more important for successful living than the factual information acquired later on.

Shouldn't the school play a part in preparing young people for marriage? Do you believe, for example, that sex education should be given in schools?

Education for marriage and parenthood should be a part of our total education, and the school should certainly play an active role in directing it along desirable channels. Instruction about sex and reproduction and about the social values of marriage and family living should be integrated into grade-school and high-school programs, in accordance, of course, with the age and the interests of the group. In colleges, courses on marriage and family life should form a prominent part of the curriculum. Several hundred colleges in the United States are already providing such courses, which are proving very helpful in giving young people basic information and an orientation about marriage and family living, and preparing them for their lives as husbands and wives and parents.

Do you advise a consultation before marriage, Doctor?

The premarital consultation, somewhat along the lines we have been following during these sessions, can be a valuable part of preparation for marriage. In ever larger numbers young people about to be married go to their physician or counselor for general or specific information about the physical and psychological aspects of marriage. Some also go to discuss specific problems which may arise before marriage. Such discussion gives them needed information and helps them to understand better their roles and functions in conjugal life. A premarital consultation lays a good foundation for the building of a successful marriage, and I would advise it whenever feasible as a routine procedure for young people about to be married.

Choice of Mate

You mentioned that you have two suggestions for the boy or girl before marriage. What is the second?

The second one is: *Choose your mate wisely.* (This, of course, no longer applies to the two of you, for you have already made your choice, and, may I say, wisely enough.) For young people contemplating marriage, the question of choice of partner is obviously of the utmost importance for the future success of their union.

In many countries the choice of a marital partner depends almost entirely on the decision of the respective families. The parents select the bride or the groom for their children, and the young couple has little choice in the matter. They may hardly even have the opportunity to become acquainted before the wedding. Among some peoples, in fact, children are betrothed while they are still very young, and later they have to marry whether they love each other or not.

In our society, however, boys and girls have the freedom to choose their own mates. This is a privilege granted by our democratic form of family organization. But freedom and privilege carry with them obligation and responsibility. If young men and women have the freedom to marry mates of their own choice, they must also have the responsibility to use insight and foresight in making their selection.

But how can one tell whether the choice is a wise one?

Attempts have been made to devise scientific tests and questionnaires to help young people to determine beforehand their degree of compatibility and their chances for success in marriage. Such tests may be useful, but only in pointing out some of the areas in which a couple may have to make a special effort to overcome probable obstacles and handicaps. There are no physical or psychological tests as yet which by themselves are a sufficient guide to the choice of a mate.

The only valid test, as I see it, is the test of time and experience. Before they marry, the boy and girl should have the time and the opportunity to become well acquainted, to be with each other under a variety of conditions, to observe each other's actions and reactions when alone and in groups, at ease and under tension, at leisure and at work, in joy and in sorrow, to learn each other's attitudes, standards and values. When two people find themselves congenial during the course of many experiences shared, there is good likelihood that their marriage will be sound and enduring.

I suppose you would advise against a hasty marriage, then?

Indeed I would. Sometimes such marriages turn out well, it is true, but the chances of success are very much lessened if the marriage is entered into on the basis of a quick romantic attachment.

Not long ago, for example, a young couple came in to see me shortly after their marriage to discuss some difficulties which had arisen in their relations. The girl had come to New York from the South three weeks before this visit. Two days after her arrival she met the man at a night club where he was performing. On the tenth day he proposed to her, and on the fifteenth day they were married. Now, five days later, they were already encountering many areas of disagreement. No bonds had been built up between them. They felt like total strangers. When I asked the husband what it was that had attracted him so violently to her the first evening, his answer was, "Well, maybe it was because she laughed so much at my jokes." But jokes oft repeated lose their freshness and their interest. Now both of them were beginning to question the wisdom of their hasty step. A night club, they found, was not an adequate place of preparation for a stable relationship.

But is not love the basic element in a happy marriage?

Yes, of course. Without a deep feeling between husband and wife no satisfactory marital relationship can develop. Without love there can be no marital happiness. It is the foundation upon which a sound companionship can be built.

The term "love," however, has many meanings. It refers not to a single emotion, but to a complexity of feelings and motivations. We may love some things or some persons because they give us pleasure, because we derive satisfaction from them. We say, for example, as Duvall and Hill point out, "I love oranges," but if the orange could talk back it might seriously question the quality of our affection. "All you want," the orange might well say, "is to squeeze the sweetness out of me and then discard me as useless." Sometimes we love people in a similar fashion, because they satisfy our needs and our desires.

Mature love involves a genuine concern for the other person's welfare. A couple maturely in love have an abiding desire to contribute to each other's physical and emotional needs, to help each other grow and develop. They "care" for each other, and they want to establish a kinship of body and of feeling. This is the kind of love on which an enduring association can be built.

Yet love alone is not enough. In our culture, at least, there is ever the possibility that the "love" we feel may be merely a romantic attachment. Romance is constantly fostered by the sentimental popular song, the magazine story, television, the press, the film, but romantic love is certainly not a sufficient basis for a lasting union. In addition to loving each other, the husband and wife should also love many things in common. They should share many interests and experiences, many attitudes and values, ideas and ideals; they should respect each other's thinking and feeling and be compatible in their general ways of life. This is the basis for a good marriage.

Suggestions for Marital Success

What suggestions would you give a couple about to marry to help them achieve a happy marriage, Doctor?

It is presumptuous for anybody even to attempt to set up specific guideposts to marital happiness, yet I might venture a few suggestions.

One: *Know thyself*. Learn about the workings of the human body, human mind, and human nature. To make a good physical adjustment, acquire knowledge of the processes of sex and reproduction; and to make a good emotional adjustment, acquire insight into your thinking and feeling. The better you know yourself, the better you will know your mate. Such knowledge leads to understanding and awareness, to tolerance and consideration, all of which are essential elements of a successful marriage.

Two: *Cherish your mate*. Marriage is a declaration of interdependence. When you marry you promise to love and to cherish each other "for better or for worse, for richer or for poorer, in sickness and in health." At the basis of your marriage is the love you bear for each other. The joy of love is the bringing of happiness to the beloved. Cherish your mate and build a strong marital tie.

A married couple are bound together by a cord, a silken cord, shall we say. This cord is made up of many strands. The strongest of these is the love and affection they bear for each other. But other strands are also necessary, the strands of mutual interests, mutual experiences, mutual loyalties, a mutual way of life. The more strands you weave into the cord, the firmer your marriage will be. Weave a strong and lasting cord, a cord that never need be severed.

Three: *When you marry, make a unit of yourselves.* "For this," says the Bible, "shall a man leave his father and his mother, and shall cleave unto his wife, and they shall be one flesh." When you marry, do not remain tied to your parents, but form a new bond with your mate. Honor thy father and thy mother, but do not cling to them. Make your own home, and give your marriage a better chance for success.

Four: *Acquire the art of physical love.* A good sexual adjustment makes a strong marital bond. Learn the techniques of love and develop a mutually satisfying physical relationship. In your togetherness, blend sentiment and sensuality. The more harmonious your sex relations are, the greater the chances for a happy marriage.

Five: *Prepare yourself for parenthood.* Acquire information about the basic facts of childbearing and child rearing. The physical and emotional well-being of your child depends largely upon the care you provide for it during its early formative years. The better you are prepared for the care of your children, the more likely they are to grow into healthy and mature adults. Till the soil well and provide a good nurture for the seed. Give your child a good start in life.

A happy home life is a good asset for any child. Children who come from happy families, from homes where the parents are affectionate, congenial and considerate, are better prepared to have a happy marriage themselves. The best preparation for parenthood is a good marriage.

Six: *Plan your family wisely.* Make a good emotional adjustment before you plan your first baby. Acquire knowledge of reliable contraceptive measures and avoid the anxieties of an unplanned conception. Children should come when they are wanted and expected. They should come by choice and not by chance.

Avoid premature parenthood, but do not delay reproduction too long. For physical and psychological reasons it is wiser to start your family early. Space your children in accordance with your needs, and plan to complete your family while both of you are still young.

Seven: *Have tolerance in your marriage.* If you dance alone you may take any steps you fancy; but if you dance with a partner, both of you must harmonize your steps. In the beginning you may step on each other's toes, but after a while, with patience and practice, you learn to adapt yourselves to each other's rhythms. In marriage too it takes time for a satisfactory physical and emotional adjustment; it takes time for two people to adapt to each other's patterns of behavior and ways of living. Tolerance and patience add to your chances for a good marriage.

Patience and tolerance are also needed by the families on both sides. It takes time for an adjustment between a new couple and the members of their respective families. Because a girl falls in love with a young man, it does not mean that she will of necessity love his mother, or that her father will necessarily like her husband. New sons- or daughters-in-law are not quickly incorporated into the inner life of another family. Time and understanding are needed for a satisfactory assimilation.

Eight: *Nurture your marriage.* Like a plant, a marriage has to be cared for and fostered, especially while it is still young. Strengthen its roots by mutual consideration, by the daily attentions and courtesies, the signs of affection and thoughtfulness, which are like the sun and the rain to make a marriage grow and flourish.

Be communicative in your expressions of affection. By word and gesture, show your feelings for each other. Love may be deeper than speech, but often it needs to be spoken. Nurture your marriage and make it grow.

The care of a plant requires also occasional weeding. If weeds are permitted to multiply, the plant may be stunted and withered. If they are removed early, the plant will have a good chance to attain its full growth. In marriage too, weed out your difficulties as they come up. Do not allow irritations to accumulate. Talk your problems over, and resolve them as they arise. Give your marriage a chance to grow and develop.

Nine: *When necessary, seek competent counsel.* If you cannot resolve your difficulties yourselves, consult an adviser. Marriage counseling is today emerging as a serious social science and social art. Physicians, ministers, social scientists, educators are training themselves for this new type of social service and practice. A trained counselor can give you understanding and insight, information and guidance, and help you prevent or remedy marital ills.

Neither of you may be aware of the hidden sources that motivate your conflicts. The cause of some disagreements may not be clear. Behind a simple argument may lie a deep sense of insecurity, or a wish for power, or a sexual frustration. If you are unable to deal with the problem yourselves, the aid of a counselor may be helpful. Seek competent guidance and further the success of your marriage.

Ten: *Follow the Golden Rule.* Do unto your mate as you would have your mate do unto you. Be aware of each other's feelings and sensitive to each other's needs. Forgive as you would be forgiven. Avoid domination or condemnation, disrespect or disloyalty, as you would have your mate avoid these toward you. This is a basic rule for all human relations, and if you adopt it also as a basic rule in your marriage relation your marriage will have an excellent chance of success.

In our culture the family is a democratic institution. It is based not on compulsion, not on binding contracts, but on binding affection and loyalty, on an inner unity and harmony between husband and wife. If you assume your mature responsibilities in your interpersonal relations, in your physical union, in planning for parenthood, in the cultivation of your marriage, your marriage will have a good chance of being both happy and successful.

Our sessions have come to an end, but your marriage journey is only at its start. During our discussions, we have charted the basic problems of the marital relation in the light of our present-day biological knowledge and social attitudes. "Married travelers," says Balzac "are in need of a pilot and a compass." Let us hope that our discussions will have served at least to point out the direction of a happy union and to guide you on the voyage to an ideal marriage.

Bibliography

This bibliography includes the books already listed after individual chapters, as well as others which have been mentioned in this volume or which have served as reference works in its preparation. In some cases, books cited or used for reference are no longer in print, but they may be found in libraries by the interested reader who wishes to consult them.

Acton, William, M.D., *The Functions and Disorders of the Reproductive Organs.* Lindsay and Blakiston, 1875.

Allen, Edgar, ed., and Young, William C., *Sex and Internal Secretions,* 3rd ed. Williams and Wilkins.

Amelar, R. D., *Infertility in Men.* Davis, 1966.

Anshen, Ruth Nanda, ed., *The Family: Its Function and Destiny,* rev. ed. Harper, 1959.

Baker, John R., *The Chemical Control of Conception.* Chapman and Hall, 1935.

Balzac, Honoré de, *The Physiology of Marriage.* Liveright, 1932. Also in Grove Press paperback.

Banning, Margaret C., *The Vine and the Olive.* Harper, 1965.

Bassett, William T., *Counseling the Childless Couple.* Prentice-Hall, 1963.

Beach, Frank A., *Hormones and Behavior,* rev. ed. Cooper Square Publishers, 1961.

Beauvoir, Simone de, *The Second Sex.* Knopf, 1953. Also in Bantam Books paperback.

Bergler, Edmund, *Counterfeit Sex: Homosexuality, Impotence, Frigidity,* 2nd rev. ed. Grove Press, 1961.

Best, Charles H., and Taylor, Norman B., *The Physiological Basis of Medical Practice.* 8th ed. Williams and Wilkins, 1966.

Blacker, C. P., M.D., *The Chances of Morbid Inheritance.* William Wood, 1934.

Bowman, Henry A., *Marriage for Moderns,* 5th ed. McGraw-Hill, 1965.

Brecher, Ruth and Edward, eds., *An Analysis of Human Sexual Response.* Signet Books, New American Library, 1966.

Briffault, Robert, *The Mothers.* Universal Library (Grosset and Dunlap), 1963.

Bromley, Dorothy D., *Catholics and Birth Control.* Devin, 1965.

Brown, Fred, and Kempton, Rudolf T., *Sex Questions and Answers: A Guide to Happy Marriage.* Whittlesey House (McGraw-Hill), 1950. Also in McGraw-Hill paperback, 1960.

Burgess, Ernest W., and Fishbein, Morris, M.D., eds., *Successful Marriage,* rev. ed. Doubleday, 1955.

——, and Locke, Harvey J., *The Family,* 3rd ed. American Book Company, 1963.

——, and others, *Courtship, Engagement and Marriage.* Lippincott, 1954.

Butterfield, Oliver M., *Sex Life in Marriage.* Emerson, 1962.

——, *Sexual Harmony in Marriage.* Emerson, 1967. Also in paperback.

Calderone, Mary S., M.D., ed., *Manual of Contraceptive Practice.* Williams and Wilkins, 1964.

Calderone, Mary S., M.D., *Release From Sexual Tensions.* Random House, 1960.

Calverton, V. E., and Schmalhausen, S. D., eds., *Sex and Civilization.* The Macaulay Company, 1929.

Capellmann, Carl, M.D., and Bergmann, W., M.D., *Pastoral Medizin.* Bonifacius Druckerei, 1923.

Carr-Saunders, A. M., *The Population Problem.* Clarendon Press, 1922.

Cavan, Ruth S., *The American Family,* 3rd ed. Crowell, 1963.

Cavanagh, John R., M.D., *Fundamental Marriage Counseling: A Catholic Viewpoint.* Bruce Publishing Company, 1963.

Christensen, Harold T., ed., *Handbook of Marriage and Family.* Rand McNally, 1964.

Clark, Le Mon, M.D., *Emotional Adjustment in Marriage.* C. V. Mosby Company, 1937.

Corner, George W., M.D., *Ourselves Unborn.* Yale University Press, 1944.

——, *The Hormones in Human Reproduction,* rev. ed. Princeton University Press, 1947.

Crawley, Ernest, *The Mystic Rose,* rev. ed. Meridian, 1960.

Davis, Katherine B., *Factors in the Sex Life of Twenty-two Hundred Women.* Harper, 1929.

Davis, Maxine, *Sexual Responsibility in Marriage.* Dial Press, 1963.

Day, Richard L., M.D., *Fertility Control: A Social Need—A Medical Responsibility.* Planned Parenthood/World Population, 1966.

Dick-Read, Grantly, M.D., *Childbirth Without Fear,* 2nd rev. ed. Harper, 1959.

——, *Natural Childbirth Primer.* Harper paperback, 1956.

Dickinson, Robert L., M.D., *The Control of Conception,* 2nd ed. Williams and Wilkins, 1938.

——, *Human Sex Anatomy,* 2nd ed. Williams and Wilkins, 1949.

——, *Techniques of Conception Control,* 3rd ed. Williams and Wilkins, 1950. Also in paperback.

——, and Beam, Laura, *Single Woman.* Williams and Wilkins, 1949.

——, *A Thousand Marriages.* Williams and Wilkins, 1931.

Dickinson, Robert L., and Gamble, Clarence J., *Human Sterilization: Techniques of Permanent Conception Control.* Human Betterment Association of America, 1950.

Duncan, J. Matthews, M.D., *Fecundity, Fertility, Sterility and Allied Topics.* Edinburgh, 1866.

Dunn, L. C., and Dobzhansky, Th., *Heredity, Race and Society.* New American Library paperback.

Durant, Will, *The Pleasures of Philosophy* (revised edition of *The Mansions of Philosophy*). Simon and Schuster, 1953. Also in paperback.

——, *The Story of Civilization,* 10v. Simon and Schuster, 1935–1967.

Duvall, Evelyn Millis, *Love and the Facts of Life.* Association Press, 1963. Also in paperback.

——, *Why Wait till Marriage?* Association Press, 1965. Also in paperback.

——, and Hill, Reuben, *When You Marry.* Association Press, 1962.

Eastman, Nicholson J., M.D., *Expectant Motherhood,* 4th rev. ed. Little, Brown, 1963.

Ellis, Havelock, *Sex and Marriage.* Random House, 1952.

——, *Studies in the Psychology of Sex,* 4v. Random House, 1925.

——, *The Psychology of Sex.* Random House, 1933; Emerson, 1938. Also in New American Library paperback.

Everett, Millard Spencer, *The Hygiene of Marriage.* Vanguard Press, 1932.

Exner, Max J., M.D., *The Sexual Side of Marriage.* Norton, 1932.

Fielding, Michael, M.D., *Parenthood–Design or Accident.* Vanguard Press, 1935.

Finegold, Wilfred J., M.D., *Artificial Insemination.* Thomas, 1964.

Fishbein, Morris, and Kennedy, R. J. R., *Modern Marriage and Family Living,* rev. ed. Doubleday, 1955.

Flanagan, Geraldine Lux, *The First Nine Months of Life.* Simon and Schuster, 1962. Also in Pocket Books paperback.

Fletcher, Joseph, *Morals and Medicine.* Beacon paperback, 1960.

Folsom, Joseph K., *The Family and Democratic Society.* Wiley, 1934.

Ford, Clellan S., *A Comparative Study of Human Reproduction.* Yale University Press, 1945.

——, and Beach, Frank A., *Patterns of Sexual Behavior.* Harper, 1951.

Forel, August, M.D., *The Sexual Question.* Physicians and Surgeons Book Company, 1931.

Freud, Sigmund, M.D., *Collected Papers,* edited by Ernest Jones, 5v. Basic Books, 1959.

——, *Basic Writings.* Modern Library, 1938.

Fromme, Allan, M.D., *Ability to Love.* Farrar, Straus, 1965. Also in Pocket Books paperback.

——, *Sex and Marriage.* Everyday Handbooks Series paperback (Barnes and Noble), 1967.

Gates, R. R., *Human Genetics,* 2v. Macmillan, 1946.

Gebhard, P. H., Pomeroy, W. W., Martin, C. E., and Christenson, C. V., *Pregnancy, Birth and Abortion.* Science Editions paperback (Wiley), 1966.

Gilbert, Margaret S., *Biography of the Unborn,* 2nd rev. ed. Hafner, 1963.

Goodrich, Frederick W., Jr., *Natural Childbirth: A Manual for Expectant Parents.* Prentice-Hall, 1950.

Gottlieb, Bernard S. and Sophie B., *What You Should Know About Marriage.* Bobbs-Merrill, 1962.

Gourmont, Rémy de, *The Natural Philosophy of Love.* Tudor (Liveright). Also in Collier paperback.

Gray, Henry, M.D., *Anatomy of the Human Body,* 28th ed., edited by C. M. Goss. Lea and Febiger, 1966.

Groves, Ernest R., *Conserving Marriage and the Family: A Realistic Discussion of the Divorce Problem.* Macmillan, 1944.

——, *Marriage.* Holt, Rinehart and Winston, 1941.

——, *Preparation for Marriage.* Emerson, 1944.

——, and others, *Sex Fulfillment in Marriage.* Emerson, 1943.

Groves, Gladys, *Marriage and Family Life.* Houghton Mifflin, 1942.

Guttmacher, Alan F., M.D., *The Case for Legalized Abortion Now.* Diablo Press, 1967.

——, *The Consumers Union Report on Family Planning,* 2nd ed. Consumers Union of the U.S., 1966.

——, *Life in the Making.* Viking Press, 1933.

——, *Pregnancy and Birth.* Signet paperback (New American Library), 1958.

——, *The Story of Human Birth.* Penguin Books, 1947.

——, with Best, Winfield, and Jaffe, Frederick S., *The Complete Book of Birth Control.* Ballantine, 1961.

Guyon, René, *The Ethics of Sexual Acts.* Knopf, 1934.

Guyot, Jules, *A Ritual for Married Lovers.* Waverly Press, 1931.

Haire, Norman, M.D., ed., *Some More Medical Views on Birth Control.* Dutton, 1928.

Haldane, J. B. S., *Daedalus, or Science and the Future.* Dutton, 1924.

Hamblen, Edwin C., M.D., *Facts for Childless Couples,* 2nd ed. Thomas, 1960.

Hamilton, G. V., M.D., *A Research in Marriage.* Albert and Charles Boni, 1929.

Hartman, Carl G., *Science and the Safe Period: A Compendium of Human Reproduction.* Williams and Wilkins, 1962.

——, *Time of Ovulation in Women.* Williams and Wilkins, 1936.

Hastings, Donald W., *Impotence and Frigidity.* Little, Brown, 1963. Also in Grove Press and Dell paperbacks.

Henry, George W., *Sex Variants.* Harper, 1941. Also in Collier paperback.

Himes, Norman E., *A Medical History of Contraception.* Gamut (Taplinger), 1964.

——, and Stone, Abraham, M.D., *Planned Parenthood—A Practical Guide to Birth Control Methods.* Collier paperback, 1964.

——, and Taylor, Donald L., *Your Marriage,* rev. ed. Holt, Rinehart and Winston, 1955.

Hirsch, E. M., *Impotence and Frigidity.* Citadel, 1966.

Hirsch, E. W., M.D., *The Power to Love.* Knopf, 1934.

Hirschfeld, Magnus, M.D., *Geschlechtskunde,* 4v. Julius Putmann, 1926.

——, *Sexual Anomalies,* rev. ed. Emerson, 1948.

Hodann, Max, M.D., *Geschlecht und Liebe.* Givelfenverlag, 1929.

——, *History of Modern Morals.* Heinemann, 1937.

Holden, Raymond T., M.D., Chairman, The Committee on Human Reproduction of the American Medical Association, "The Control of Fertility," *Journal of the American Medical Association,* Vol. 194, pp. 462–470 (Oct. 25, 1965).

Holmes, John Haynes, *Marriage and Happiness*. The Community Church, 1930.

Hotchkiss, Robert S., M.D., *Fertility in Men*. Lippincott, 1944.

Huhner, Max, M.D., *Disorders of the Sexual Function in the Male and Female*. F. A. Davis Company, 1920.

Huntington, Ellsworth, *Tomorrow's Children*. Wiley, 1935.

Isaac, Rael Jean, *Adopting a Child Today*. Harper and Row, 1965.

Jarcho, Julius, M.D., *Postures and Practices during Labor among Primitive Peoples*. Paul B. Hoeber, 1934.

Jennings, H. S., *The Biological Basis of Human Nature*. Norton, 1930.

Kahn, Fritz, M.D., *Our Sex Life*. Knopf, 1945.

Kaufman, Sherwin A., M.D., *The Ageless Woman*. Prentice-Hall, 1967.

Kinsey, Alfred C., and others, *Sexual Behavior in the Human Female*. Saunders, 1953. Also in Pocket Books paperback.

——, Pomeroy, W. B., and Martin, Clyde E., *Sexual Behavior in the Human Male*. Saunders, 1948.

Kisch, E. Heinrich, M.D., *The Sexual Life of Woman*. Allied Book Company, 1931.

Kleegman, Sophie J., and Kaufman, S. A., *Infertility in Women*. Davis, 1966.

Knaus, Herman, M.D., *Human Procreation and Its Natural Regulation*. Obolensky, 1963.

Knowlton, Charles, M.D., *The Fruits of Philosophy*. Pauper Press, 1937.

Kopp, Marie E., *Birth Control in Practice*. Robert McBride and Company, 1934.

Lader, Lawrence, *Abortion*. Bobbs-Merrill, 1966.

Landis, Judson T. and Mary G., *Building a Successful Marriage*, 4th ed. Prentice-Hall, 1963.

——, *Personal Adjustment, Marriage and Family Living*, 4th ed. Prentice-Hall, 1966.

Landman, J. H., *Human Sterilization*. Macmillan, 1932.

Latz, Leo J., M.D., *The Rhythm of Sterility and Fertility in Women*. Latz Foundation, 1939.

Lerrigo, Marion O., and Southard, Helen, *The Story About You: The Facts You Want to Know About Sex*. Dutton, 1956.

——, *What's Happening to Me? Sex Education for the Teenager*. Dutton, 1956.

Leslie, Gerald R., *The Family in Social Context*. Oxford University Press, 1967.

Leuba, Clarence, *Ethics in Sex Conduct*. Association Press, 1948.

Levy, John, M.D., and Munroe, Ruth, *The Happy Family*. Knopf, 1938. Also in paperback.

Lindsay, Judge Ben B., and Evans, Wainwright, *The Companionate Marriage*. Garden City Publishing Company, 1929.

Locke, Harvey J., *Predicting Adjustment in Marriage*. Holt, Rinehart and Winston, 1951.

Loeb, Jacques, *The Organism as a Whole*. Putnam, 1916.

Long, H. W., M.D., *Sane Sex Life and Sane Sex Living*. Richard G. Badger, 1919.

Lydston, G. Frank, M.D., *Impotence and Sterility*. The Riverton Press, 1917.

Malinowski, Bronislaw, *The Sexual Life of Savages in Northwestern Melanesia.* Harcourt, Brace and World, paperback, 1962.

Mantegazza, Paolo, *Sexual Relations of Mankind.* Wehman. Also in Parliament paperback.

Marshall, F. H. A., and Parkes, A. S., *The Physiology of Reproduction.* 3rd ed., 3v. Little, Brown. Vol. 1, Part 1, 1956; Part 2, 1960; Vol. 2, 1961; Vol. 3, 1965.

Masters, W. H., and Johnson, V. E., *Human Sexual Response.* Little, Brown, 1966.

May, Geoffrey, *Social Control of Sex Expression.* William Morrow, 1930.

Mead, Margaret, *Coming of Age in Samoa.* Modern Library, 1953. Also in Dell paperback.

——, *Male and Female: A Study of the Sexes in a Changing World.* William Morrow, 1949.

Meaker, Samuel R., M.D., *Human Sterility.* Williams and Wilkins, 1934.

Merrill, Francis E., *Society and Culture,* 3rd ed. Prentice-Hall, 1965.

Metchnikoff, Elie, *The Nature of Man.* Putnam, 1903.

Moench, Gerard L., M.D., *Studien zur Fertilität.* Enke, 1931.

Moll, Albert, *The Sexual Life of the Child.* Macmillan, 1923.

Montagu, M. F. Ashley, *Adolescent Sterility.* Thomas, 1946.

Moore, Carl R., "The Biology of the Testis," in *Sex and Internal Secretions.* Williams and Wilkins, 1939.

Muller, H. J., *Out of the Night.* Vanguard Press, 1935.

Nafzawi, Umar Ibn Muhammad Al, *The Perfumed Garden.* Privately printed.

Naismith, Grace, *Private and Personal.* McKay, 1966.

Neubardt, Selig, *A Concept of Contraception.* Trident Press (Pocket Books), 1967.

Nimkoff, Meyer F., *Marriage and the Family.* Houghton Mifflin, 1947.

Noyes, Humphrey John, *Male Continence.* Oneida, 1870.

Ogino, Kyusaku, M.D., *Conception Period of Women.* Medical Arts Publishing Company, 1934.

Osborn, Frederick, *Preface to Eugenics.* Harper, 1940.

Ovid, *Ars Amatoria.* Privately printed.

Papanicolaou, George N., "The Sexual Cycle in the Human Female as Revealed by Vaginal Smears," *The American Journal of Anatomy,* May 1933.

Parshley, H. M., *The Science of Human Reproduction.* Norton, 1933.

Peterson, James A., *Toward a Successful Marriage.* Scribner's, 1960.

Pincus, Gregory, *The Eggs of Mammals.* Macmillan, 1936.

Ploscowe, Morris, *Sex and the Law.* Prentice-Hall, 1951.

Ploss, Heinrich, and Bartels, Max and Paul, *Woman,* 3v. C. V. Mosby Company, 1938.

Popenoe, Paul, *The Child's Heredity.* Williams and Wilkins, 1929.

Portnoy, Louise, and Saltman, Jules, *Fertility in Marriage: A Guide for the Childless.* Collier paperback, 1962.

Power, Jules, *How Life Begins.* Simon and Schuster, 1965.

Rainer, Jerome and Julia, *Sexual Pleasure in Marriage.* Simon and Schuster, 1959.

Reynolds, Edward, M.D., and Macomber, Donald, M.D., *Fertility and Sterility in Human Marriages*. Saunders, 1924.

Robie, W. F., M.D., *The Art of Love*. Brown, 1962. Also in Parliament paperback.

Robinson, William J., M.D., *Sexual Impotence*. Eugenics Publishing Company, 1933.

Robinson, J. F., *Having a Baby*, 3rd ed. Williams and Wilkins, 1966.

Rock, John, M.D., *The Time Has Come*. Knopf, 1963.

Rock, John, M.D., and Loth, David, *Voluntary Parenthood*. Random House, 1949.

Russell, Bertrand, *Marriage and Morals*. Liveright, 1929.

St. John-Stevas, Norman, *Right to Life*. Holt, Rinehart and Winston, 1964.

Sanger, Margaret, *An Autobiography*. Norton, 1938.

——, *Happiness in Marriage*. Coward-McCann, 1926.

——, *Motherhood in Bondage*. Coward-McCann, 1928.

——, ed., *Biological and Medical Aspects of Contraception*. National Committee on Federal Legislation for Birth Control, 1934.

——, and Stone, Hannah M., M.D., eds., *The Practice of Contraception*. Williams and Wilkins, 1931.

Scheinfeld, Amram, *Your Heredity and Environment* (formerly *The New You and Heredity*). Lippincott, 1965.

——, *Women and Men*. Harcourt, Brace, 1943.

Schur, Edwin M., ed., *The Family and the Sexual Revolution: Selected Readings*. Indiana University Press, 1964.

Seward, Georgene H., *Sex and the Social Order*. McGraw-Hill, 1946.

Siegler, Samuel L., M.D., *Fertility in Women*. Lippincott, 1944.

Smith, David T., ed., *Abortion and the Law*. Press of Western Reserve University, 1967.

Snyder, Laurence H., *Medical Genetics*. Duke University Press, 1941.

Spallanzani, Lazarro, *Dissertations*, 2v. 1784.

Steinach, Eugen, M.D., *Sex and Life*. Viking Press, 1940.

Stekel, Wilhelm, M.D., *Frigidity in Woman*. Liveright, 1962. Also in Grove Press paperback, 2v.

——, *Impotence in the Male*, 2v., rev. ed. Liveright, 1955. Also Black Cat paperback (Grove Press), 2v. 1965.

Stockham, Alice B., M.D., *Karezza—Ethics of Marriage*. R. F. Fenno, 1903.

Stone, Abraham, M.D., "Coitus Interruptus," in *The Practice of Contraception*, edited by Margaret Sanger and Hannah M. Stone. Williams and Wilkins, 1931.

——, "How Can We Have a Baby?," *Redbook* magazine, May 1954.

——, and Levine, Lena, *Premarital Consultation*. Grune, 1956.

Stone, Hannah M., M.D., "Birth Control as a Factor in the Sex Life of Women," in *Sexual Reform Congress*. 1930.

——, *Maternal Health and Contraception*. Maternal Health Center, Newark, New Jersey, 1933.

——, and Stone, Abraham, M.D., "Marital Maladjustments," in *Cyclopedia of Medicine, Surgery and Specialties*. F. A. Davis, 1945.

Stopes, Marie C., *Married Love*. Putnam, 1929.

——, *Contraception*. Putnam, 1931.

Suenens, Leon J., *Love and Control.* Newman, 1961.

Taussig, Frederick J., M.D., "Abortion Control through Birth Control," in *Biological and Medical Aspects of Contraception.* 1934.

——, *Abortion, Spontaneous and Induced.* C. V. Mosby, 1936.

Terman, Lewis M., *Psychological Factors in Marital Happiness.* McGraw-Hill, 1938.

Thomas, John L., S.J., *Looking toward Marriage.* Fides Publishers, 1964.

——, *Marriage and Rhythm.* Newman, 1957.

Trainer, Joseph B., *Physiologic Foundations for Marriage Counseling.* Mosby, 1965.

Truxal, Andrew C., and Merrill, Francis E., *The Family in American Culture.* Prentice-Hall, 1947.

Tushnov, M. P., M.D., *Spermatoxins.* Kazan, 1911.

Van de Velde, T. H., M.D., *Ideal Marriage,* rev. ed. Random House, 1965.

——, *Fertility and Sterility in Marriage.* Random House, 1931.

Vatsyayana, *The Kama Sutra.* Putnam paperback, 1963.

Voge, Cecil L. B., *The Chemistry and Physics of Contraceptives.* Jonathan Cape, 1933.

Voronoff, Serge, M.D., *The Conquest of Life.* Coward-McCann, 1928.

Watson, John, *Behaviorism.* University of Chicago Press, 1958. Also in Phoenix paperback.

Weisman, Abner I., M.D., *Spermatozoa and Sterility.* Paul B. Hoeber, 1941.

Weiss, Edward, M.D., and English, O. Spurgeon, M.D., *Psychosomatic Medicine,* 3rd ed. Saunders, 1957.

Westermarck, Edward, *The History of Human Marriage,* 3v. Macmillan, 1922.

——, *Short History of Marriage.* College Library, 1926.

Wile, Ira S., M.D., ed., *The Sex Life of the Unmarried Adult.* Vanguard Press, 1934.

Williams, Glanville, *The Sanctity of Life and the Criminal Law.* Knopf, 1957.

Williams, J. Whitridge, M.D., *Obstetrics.* Appleton-Century Company, 1926.

Woodbury, Robert Morse, *Causal Factors in Infant Mortality.* Children's Bureau Publication No. 142, U.S. Department of Labor, 1925.

Wright, Helena, M.D., *The Sex Factor in Marriage.* Vanguard Press, 1931.

Young, William C., *Sex and Internal Secretions,* 3rd ed. Williams and Wilkins. 1961.

Zuckerman, S., *The Social Life of Monkeys and Apes.* Harcourt, Brace and Company, 1932.

Index

Abdomen, 42, 64
    enlargement of, during pregnancy, 101
Abortions:
    danger of, 174
    definition of, 202
    indications for, 202
    in Japan, 176
    legal, 173
    measures for control of, 203
    miscarriages and, 202
    nature of, 202
    among primitive peoples, 124
    reasons for, 202–203
    in Scandinavia, 176
    in Soviet Union, 175–176
    therapeutic indications for, 173, 176–177, 202
    in U.S., 173
Abstinence, sexual (*see* Continence, sexual)
Accessory male sex glands (*see* Male sex organs)
Acton, William, 219
Adrenal glands, 57
Afterbirth (*see* Placenta)
Age:
    fertility and, 180–182
    marriage and, 271–273, 274, 291–292
    of maturity, 271, 273–274
    of menopause, 75, 180
    of puberty, 180
    reproduction and, 273–274
Allen, Edgar, 71
Anatomy:
    of female sex organs, 63–89
    of male sex organs, 41–61
    of sexual intercourse, 77–82, 212–214
Anesthesia:
    during childbirth, 110
    during surgical defloration, 216
Animals:
    artificial fertilization, 199–200
    artificial insemination, 194–195
    breeding capacity, 179
    castration, 58, 86
    courtship, 220–221
    gland transplantation, 59–60
    "heat" period, 283
    modes of reproduction, 91–93
    periodicity of sexual desire, 283–284
Anxiety neurosis (*see* Fears and anxieties)
Art of love, 209–212, 221–224, 227, 246–247, 317
Art of marriage, 207–234, 316–319
Artificial fertilization, 198–201
Artificial insemination, 194–201
    in animals, 194–195
    in humans, 194–197
    legality of, 197–198
    purpose of, 196
Aschheim-Zondek test for pregnancy, 102
Asexual reproduction, 92
Autoerotism (*see* Masturbation)
Azoospermia:
    causes of, 186
    definition of, 185
    frequency of, 186
    sterility and, 185, 186
    test to determine, 186–187

Bag of waters, 108
Balzac, Honoré de, 211, 221, 235, 319
Barrenness (*see* Infertility)
Bartels, 215
Bartholin's gland, 83, 212, 224
Beach, Frank A., 231, 262
Beam, Laura, 208
Behaviorism, 27

Fitness for marriage (cont'd)
    emotional, 19–20
    eugenic, 21–27
    health and, 23–24
    reproductive, 21–22
    sexual, 21
    standards of, 16
Foam creams, 144–145, 153
Follicle (see Ovulation)
Ford, Clellan S., 231, 262, 285
Foreskin of penis, 50–52
    circumcision, 51–52
Forceps, 111
Freud, Sigmund, 209, 290
Frigidity, sexual, 242–248, 257 (see
    also Sexual adjustments and
    maladjustments)
    case histories, 245, 257
    causes of, 242–248, 259–261
    degrees of, 242–243
    in female, 242–243
    frequency of, 243
    in male, 256–257
    treatment of, 246–248
Fructose, 48

Galen, 233
Galton, Francis, 37
Genes, 26–27, 54, 68, 92 (see also
    Chromosomes; Heredity)
Genital disproportion:
    case history, 261–262
    sexual adjustment and, 260–261
Genital organs (see Female sex or-
    gans; Male sex organs)
Genital spasm, 238–241
    case history, 238–239
    as cause of sexual disharmonies,
    239
    causes of, 238–241
    treatment of, 241
Genital system (see Female sex or-
    gans; Male sex organs)
Genital tract (see Female sex organs;
    Male sex organs)
Germ cells (see Sex cells)
German measles:
    congenital defects and, 28

Glands (see also separate listing for
    each gland)
    adrenal glands, 57
    Bartholin's glands, 83, 212, 224
    mammary glands, 58, 85, 103,
    114–115, 222
    pituitary gland, 46, 57, 64, 86,
    107
    secretions of (see Hormones)
    sex glands, 44, 57, 58, 64
    thyroid gland, 57
    urethral glands, 52
Gland transplantation:
    in animals, 59–60, 87
    of female gland into male, 87
    in humans, 60, 87–88
    of male gland into female, 59–60
Glandular disturbances:
    as cause of azoospermia, 185
    as cause of frigidity, 259
    as cause of impotence, 260
    as cause of sterility, 185
    homosexuality and, 266
Glans of penis, 50
Golden rule, in marital happiness,
    319
Gonads (see Sex glands)
Gonorrhea: (see also Venereal dis-
    eases)
    as cause of blindness in the new-
    born, 32
    as cause of prostate disease, 49
    as cause of sterility, 48, 185
    curability of, 33
    heredity and, 31–32
    transmissibility of, 32, 34
Graafian follicle, 66
Groves, Ernest R., 298
Guttmacher, Alan Frank, 72
Guyot, Jean, 217

Hair:
    pubic hair, 79
    as sexual character, 57–58
Haldane, J. B. S., 201
Hall, R. E., 149
Hamilton, G. V., 249
Happiness in marriage, 126, 233, 235–
    236, 276, 293–295, 297–319

ABOUT THE AUTHORS

Dr. Hannah Stone was a medical pioneer in the birth-control movement in America, and for nearly two decades she was associated with Margaret Sanger as Medical Director of the Margaret Sanger Research Bureau in New York. With Dr. Abraham Stone she founded the first Marriage Consultation Center in America, which was located first at the Labor Temple and later at the Community Church in New York. She lectured widely on the subjects of marriage, the family, and birth control, and her articles appeared in many medical and scientific journals. With Margaret Sanger she edited The Prevention of Conception, *a pioneer volume on the subject, and was a member of the Editorial Advisory Board of the* Journal of Human Fertility. *Dr. Hannah Stone died in July 1941.*

Dr. Abraham Stone was the Medical Director of the Marriage Consultation Center of the Community Church, and former president of the American Association of Marriage Counselors. In 1947 he was given the Lasker Award for his contributions to marriage counseling and planned parenthood.

He was also the Director of the Margaret Sanger Research Bureau and a vice-president of the Planned Parenthood Federation of America. For thirteen years he was the editor of the Journal of Human Fertility, *and was then a member of the editorial board of the journal* Fertility and Sterility *and also of* Marriage and Family Living. *With Dr. Norman Hine he wrote the book* Planned Parenthood.

He was also on the faculty of the New School for Social Research, directing the course dealing with Marriage and Family Living and Marriage Counseling. In addition, he was a member of the faculty of the New York University College of Medicine. Dr. Abraham Stone died in August 1959 at the age of 69.